Radiation Therapy
of Tumors and Diseases
of the Nervous System

JEAN BOUCHARD, M.D., F.A.C.R., F.R.C.P.(C)

Professor of Radiology, McGill University
Consultant in Radiation Therapy, Montreal Neurological Hospital
Chief, Department of Therapeutic Radiology, Royal Victoria Hospital
Montreal, Canada

Lea & Febiger

Philadelphia   1966

foreword

MODERN neurosurgery in the early stages of its development was mainly concerned with the treatment of patients with brain tumors. Almost from the beginning radiation therapy was utilized in the sizeable proportion of patients whose tumors either could not be completely removed, or showed a strong tendency to recur despite apparently complete removal. The scope of the field of neurosurgery has increased markedly during the past 50 years or so, but neoplasms of the central nervous system continue to provide the neurosurgeon with some of his most challenging problems. The percentage of these patients who can be cured by surgery alone has not increased significantly despite the precise diagnostic tools and the improved surgical and anesthetic techniques now available, and the earlier referral of patients for definitive treatment. As radiation techniques and equipment have improved, the role of radiation therapy has steadily expanded in the treatment of many types of central nervous system neoplasms.

Close co-operation between the neurologist or neurosurgeon and the radiation therapist is essential if patients with neoplasms of the central nervous system are to derive maximum benefit from surgery and irradiation, the only two potent weapons in our therapeutic resources at present. Since the opening of the Montreal Neurological Institute in 1934 a close and harmonious collaborative program has existed between the Radiation Therapy Department of the Royal Victoria Hospital and the Montreal Neurological Institute (which also constitutes the Department of Neurology and Neurosurgery of the Royal Victoria Hospital). I speak for the co-founders of the Institute, Dr. Wilder Penfield and the late Dr. William V. Cone, as well as for all its senior staff members, in expressing the great debt of gratitude we owe Dr. Jean Bouchard for his enthusiastic co-operation and for his expert, meticulous and thoughtful work in providing maximally effective and safe radiation therapy for our patients with neoplasms and other lesions of the nervous system.

Energetic and persistent efforts by Dr. Bouchard and his staff, in their series of 564 consecutive patients with primary brain tumors who received an adequate course of irradiation between 1939 and 1958 inclusive, have resulted in complete follow-up data of 5 to 25 years' duration on all but one patient, and he was lost to follow-up only after a period of 17 years. These data, which form the backbone of this monograph, constitute a unique body of information because of completeness, duration of follow-up and accuracy. Hence this monograph will serve as a reference work of special interest and value to neurologists, neurosurgeons and other clinicians concerned with the care of patients with neoplasms of the nervous system.

Radiologists will be equally interested in the chapters summarizing our present knowledge of radiation effects on the nervous system, the present role of irradiation in the treatment of the various types of tumors of the central and peripheral nervous system, and in the lucid descriptions of the radiation techniques developed and employed by Dr. Bouchard.

THEODORE RASMUSSEN, M.D.
Professor of Neurology and Neurosurgery, McGill University
Director, Montreal Neurological Institute and Hospital
Montreal, Canada

preface

My INTENTION in writing this book was to prepare a comprehensive review of all the essential facts necessary for the understanding and sound clinical approach to the treatment of lesions of the central nervous system. This has been accomplished to the best of my ability for all those, including therapeutic radiologists, who may be interested in the management of patients affected primarily with neoplastic lesions and occasionally other diseases of the nervous system. In this volume, one will find that the emphasis has been placed on the evaluation of the most recent advances and progress of radiation therapy in this field, in addition to a presentation of radiotherapeutic techniques.

Twenty-four years ago, Dyke and Davidoff wrote a monograph entitled *Roentgen Treatment of Diseases of the Nervous System*. The volume was approximately the same size as this and the publishers were also Lea & Febiger. Dyke and Davidoff contributed considerably to my guidance and that of many others in this particular aspect of radiotherapeutics. Their fine work, to my knowledge, has remained the sole of the kind, at least in the English medical literature.

In response to a need identical to that felt by my predecessors, I am endeavoring to re-evaluate the role of radiation therapy today in the management of tumors and diseases of the nervous system. Some experimental data have brought confusion in minds because of conditions of irradiation often excessive in comparison with tissue tolerance in clinical usage. The need is great for practical information regarding radiobiological effects on the central nervous tissues and tumors, in relation to clinical therapeutic applications. The potential hazard of post-irradiation injury and the contributing factors must be reviewed, analyzed and digested. Long-term treatment results were required for that type of evaluation. Such have become available, proving to be highly informative, stimulating and encouraging.

A glance at the table of contents should quickly enable one to visualize the broad scope covered in this volume. It is hoped that this text may serve as a source of reference for all those concerned with the treatment of lesions, particularly tumors, affecting the intracranial and intraspinal content. Undergraduate and postgraduate students, specialists in neurology, neurosurgery, radiology and other fields of medical endeavor may find under one cover answers to many questions coming to their minds.

The first three chapters contain a considerable amount of basic information deemed essential to the understanding and sound approach to most problems related to the treatment of lesions of the central nervous system. The effect of radiation therapy, immediate and remote, must be reviewed and re-assessed for all patients exposed to irradiation used alone or as part of treatment for tumors of the central nervous system. Long-term results have been presented on the basis of survival and recovery rates side by side, following re-assessment every 5-year period among those who survived over 5, 10, 15, or 20 years subsequent to irradiation. When considering the overall picture, I feel justified to state that such results are encouraging.

A substantial part of this book deals with the primary intracranial gliomas in which the role of surgical management is predominant. Each histological type of intracranial gliomas has been discussed and the part of radiation therapy reviewed in the treatment of primary tumors and recurrences, by comparison with identical series of non-irradiated patients. The effect of radiation therapy alone in the management of mid-brain and brain stem tumors may astonish many, in a group of patients considered to have a rather poor prognosis.

The treatment of non-gliomatous primary intracranial neoplasms is largely a surgical problem. The extent to which irradiation may be useful in the management of some of them has also been reviewed.

There is a need for information regarding the late results of treatment in infants and children exposed to intensive irradiation during the period of somatic and mental development. Our long-term results over 5 to 20 years or longer, following treatment given at the age of 15 or less for tumors affecting the mid-brain and brain stem, medulloblastomas or cerebellar sarcomas, or other tumors, are provided in a separate chapter.

The management of tumors of the pituitary gland deserves a special look. This is particularly necessary as our concepts of endocrine functions of this gland are in continuous evolution. We feel that this subject could not be discussed without some reference to the physio-pathological changes which may allow for some evaluation of the influence of radiation therapy in the treatment of pituitary tumors.

Our text would not be complete without considering the effects of radiation in the palliation of metastatic intracranial tumors, its influence on spinal cord tumors and other lesions. The limited role that radiation therapy may play in the management of certain lesions involving the peripheral nervous system has been outlined.

In writing this volume, I have tried to bring an objective approach in the discussion of the indications for treatment and the selection of the methods available, whether surgical, radiological, or chemotherapeutic, used alone or in combination. This has been attempted without prejudice for or against any given method of treatment by presenting as factual information as could be gathered. It was not feasible to review the work of and give credit to more workers in this special field, and I hope there will be no offence.

There is a dictum that nothing succeeds as success, and very little is more depressing and discouraging than failure. In relation to the efficacy of a method of treatment, the particular case which for better or for worse remains vivid in our minds as a perpetual evocation must not influence and guide indefinitely our therapeutic efforts and teaching. An overall picture allows a broader perspective, so that greater wisdom may prevail in the clinical judgment of individual cases. I sincerely hope that this book will serve that purpose by conveying the most complete and up to the moment information available.

I wish to express my deep appreciation to the entire Staff of the Montreal Neurological Institute who through the years have contributed in so many ways to the results presented here. It is through their valuable assistance and moral support that we have been able together to pursue this clinical work. I must pay tribute to my outstanding colleagues, in particular Drs. W. Penfield, T. Rasmussen, A. Elvidge, and the late W. Cone. I am indebted also to my fellow radiologists, Drs. C. B. Peirce and D. L. McRae.

I owe Dr. T. Rasmussen, Director of the Montreal Neurological Institute and Hospital, a special expression of deep appreciation for gracefully writing a foreword to this book.

It is proper to acknowledge the obligingness of Dr. Gilbert Fletcher, Director of the M. D. Anderson Tumor Institute at the University of Texas, for his support in promoting the publication of this monograph. I must thank him for allowing me to use some of my own material already published under his editorship in a *Textbook of Radiation Therapy* (1966).

My devoted secretary, Mrs. Agnes Boudreau, deserves my sincere gratitude. It is largely due to her dedication over the last 12 years that the follow-up of our patients is so complete. Her assistance in the final editing of this book has been splendid. I also wish to express my appreciation to my secretarial assistant, Mrs. Barbara Glavicich. Our medical artist, Mrs. Judith Gebhard Smith, has contributed much in providing attractive illustrations. Dr. G. Mathieson has been most helpful in re-classifying some cases with pathologic diagnoses rarely used nowadays; and also in the preparation of the neuro-pathologic material included in our illustrations.

Finally, I acknowledge the co-operation of all members of my Staff, including our radiation physicists and radiological technicians, present and past, for their indefatigable assistance.

JEAN BOUCHARD
Montreal, Canada

Contents

Introduction

THE USE of ionizing radiation and high energy ionizing particles is a valid method of treatment in the management of tumors of the central nervous system, either primary or metastatic. Radiation therapy may be efficacious also in a few selected lesions affecting the peripheral nervous system.

It should be stated from the onset of this monograph that adequate irradiation of tumors involving the brain or other intracranial structures, the pons, and the spinal cord can be accomplished with minimal risks of damage to the adjacent tissues and intervening normal anatomical structures. The beneficial effects of radiation therapy in the management of lesions of the central and peripheral nervous system have been considerably greater, in our experience, than the rare actual or potential adverse effects. Such observation is also relevant to the use of radiation therapy in pituitary tumors. It is valid not only for adults but for infants and children as well.

Analysis of our long-term results has demonstrated that the length and quality of survival of patients irradiated in the treatment of most types of primary intracranial neoplasms are generally better than expected. It has also proved that children affected with malignant brain tumors can be exposed to intensive irradiation without significant risk of undue physical or mental sequelae. Radiation therapy can be and often is of considerable value as a palliative measure against cerebral metastases.

In pituitary tumors, irradiation alone has arrested tumor growth over long periods of time.

Irradiation of primary tumors of the spinal cord appears to be of definite value although it is sometimes difficult to assess. It is a very effective therapeutic measure in the treatment of most of the extradural tumors pressing on the cord. The controversial usefulness of radiation in the treatment of non-neoplastic conditions such as syringomyelia and arachnoiditis will be discussed.

In the last chapter of this monograph a brief reference will be made regarding the role of radiation therapy in the management of neoplastic and non-neoplastic diseases affecting the peripheral nervous system including the cranial nerves. Consideration will be given to the value of radiation therapy for the relief of pain in neuritis and neuralgia, or pain and pruritus when associated with scars and keloids. The analgesic effect of irradiation is of paramount importance in the control of pain related to primary or metastatic neoplastic manifestations involving nerve roots, trunks or endings, or else affecting visceral and skeletal structures.

The role of radiation therapy in the management of lesions involving the nervous system will be discussed fully for each pathologic condition. The value of irradiation, whether used in combination with surgical procedures or alone, will be assessed by comparison with other modes of treatment, on the basis of the immediate and late clinical results observed and reported.

Primary Intracranial Neoplasms:
General Considerations

PRIMARY INTRACRANIAL NEOPLASMS represent today a group of neoplastic manifestations which, despite their growth in a vital area controlling all mental and somatic functions, can be and should be treated with enough efficacy as to yield a relatively large proportion of long survivals and high recovery rates. This situation has resulted from a number of favorable factors related to the natural history of such tumors, the extreme degree of precision attained in their localization and diagnosis, and the efficacy of therapeutic measures applicable to them.

NATURAL HISTORY AND SPECIAL CHARACTERISTICS

Certain natural factors, peculiar to primary intracranial neoplasms, must be emphasized so that their significance be fully appreciated in the management of such tumors. It is important to realize that the growth and extension of the majority of primary intracranial tumors is essentially a localized and regional neoplastic process from beginning to end. Only a small proportion of those tumors ever extend beyond the cranial cavity, and when extension does occur it is nearly always into the spinal canal or the cord. The natural tendency that most primary intracranial tumors have to remain localized should be regarded as a favorable factor in their treatment. It clearly indicates that the biologic and histopathologic characters of many of those tumors are rather benign in their neoplastic behavior. However, even when their histopathologic characteristics are not malignant, primary intracranial tumors are ordinarily considered malignant because they are capable of causing death. Such malignant potentiality is in a large measure attributable to their anatomic location.

The lack of anatomical space to expand within the rigid cranial cavity is mainly responsible for the profound mechanical disturbances which may result from the growth of an intracranial tumor. The extent to which tumor growth is interfering with circulation of the cerebrospinal fluid will partly determine the degree of increased intracranial pressure which may affect at once the entire brain and its various components. The incidence of generalized intracranial edema and the degree of severity of symptoms are directly related to and commensurate with the over-all increase of intracranial pressure. As the tumor grows intracranially it also exerts direct local and regional pressure on the adjacent normal nervous tissue, disturbing its normal functions and causing various neurological signs. Disturbances in the blood circulation occur at least at the site of the tumor and localized edema is often observed at the same time at its periphery. Occasionally, secondary cystic gliosis and sometimes necrosis may be observed. The tumor by its growth may also cause pressure upon cranial nerves which may become atrophied. The existence of such tissue reactions and complications, primarily caused by the tumor growth, must be recognized when present. Too often such reactions are ignored as initial manifestations of intracranial tumors and are subsequently attributed to the surgical or radiotherapeutic treatment employed to control the intracranial neoplasm itself.

A very significant anatomical factor in keeping most of the primary intracranial tumors within the cranial cavity is the absence of lymphatic channels in the central nervous system. The possibility of dissemination of tumor cells by lymphatics to other parts of the body does not exist in brain tumors. This is a rare and highly favorable feature in the treatment of neoplastic conditions.

Spontaneous dissemination of primary brain tumors through the blood stream appears to be extremely uncommon. In the rare cases in which human gliomas have been found in the lungs and other viscera at autopsy Zimmerman[126] believes that such tumors "seem to have metastasized to these locations following a surgical attack upon them". Cerebral blood vessels present a major barrier to distant dissemination of primary brain tumors in resisting invasion of their lumen by tumor cells. The nature of this phenomenon would seem to be more biologic than anatomic. It has been studied extensively by a few neuropathologists, particularly by Zimmerman[126] who has produced experimental gliomas in hundreds of mice and has not observed a single case of spontaneous extracranial metastasis. He has concluded that gliogenous tumor cells are unable to invade cerebral blood vessels. More recently (1962), Luse,[71] in her electron microscopic studies of brain tumors, has reported that she has never seen a glial cell in the center of a blood vessel, even when glial cells could be seen within the adventitia of the vessel.

The only natural anatomical avenue of dissemination for tumor cells detached from primary intracranial neoplasms is along the subarachnoid spaces where cerebrospinal fluid is circulating. This mode of spread seems to occur spontaneously mostly in medulloblastomas, and occasionally in the less common ependymoblastomas and sarcomas of the brain. The tumor implants, which may result from such shedding of cells by the primary tumor, are usually found first distally to the tumor itself in the direction of the cerebrospinal fluid flow along the spinal axis. However, once the cerebrospinal flow is blocked by the tumor it may reverse its direction so that circulating tumor cells can ascend into the ventricles and the subarachnoid spaces around the cerebral hemispheres. This is an adverse factor which must be taken into serious account in the management and treatment of tumors in which it occurs.

Artificial avenues of dissemination of tumor cells may result from the use of shunts in deviating the cerebrospinal flow for controlling increased intracranial pressure. At autopsy, a large peritoneal implant, surrounding the end of a ventriculo-peritoneal shunt was found in one of our patients, who also had other distant metastases from a primary cerebellar sarcoma. It is reasonable to assume that ventriculo-atrial shunts might spread tumor cells through the bloodstream and contribute to increase the incidence of heretofore rare extracranial metastases. Viable cells from experimentally induced ependymoma have been injected into the jugular veins of mice by Kageyama,[50] who has observed metastases in only 9 of 42 mice, all to the lung and none to any other organ. In humans, in the event of dissemination through the bloodstream by a shunt or other surgical procedures, immunological reactions presumably could prevent survival and reproduction of cells from gliomas or other primary intracranial neoplasms in most cases.

Tumor implants in operative wounds or scars are extremely rare following removal of even the most malignant intracranial neoplasms. We have yet to observe a single direct surgical transplantation of human glioma arising from an operative scar. That is in contrast with the incidence of tumor implants observed in scars following surgical removal of malignancies from other organs in the human body. Contrary to the experience with human gliomas, Zimmerman[126] has successfully transplanted animal gliomas extracranially in almost 100 per cent of trials in the mouse, by direct implant into brain, eyes, liver, kidney, peritoneum and subcutaneous tissue. The above differences between clinical and experimental tumor transplant behavior might be explained by immunological factors or other biological incompatibility between cell and host tissue.

The natural tendency that most primary brain tumors have to remain localized intracranially has been explained above with histopathologic, anatomic and biologic facts. It is essential also that their intracranial behavior be clearly known and understood. The gliomas, which represent approximately 50 per cent of all primary intracranial tumors, usually grow as a single tumor mass but may be multicentric and form more than one tumor when they originate simultaneously either in one or in both cerebral hemispheres, or in some other anatomic part of the central nervous tissue.

Infiltrating types of gliomatous tumors may extend to the opposite side of the brain under the falx cerebri through the corpus callosum, a finding which is not too unusual when one is aware of this and seeks for it. Infiltrating gliomas may also extend down into the brainstem or the basal ganglia, or else they may originate in the brainstem and extend upwards into the mid-brain and beyond, in either way always by direct neoplastic invasion of the adjacent central nervous structures. Such modalities of the growth and intracranial extension of primary brain tumors must be known and identified when present, lest the treatment applied be inadequate because part of the extension of the new growth has been ignored.

It was stated above that only a small proportion of primary intracranial neoplasms ever extend directly beyond the cranial cavity. Meningeal tumors may occasionally extend directly through the dura and calvarium under the scalp or through the base of the skull into adjacent cavities. Chordomas and craniopharyngiomas also extend at times directly outside of the cranial cavity proper into the sphenoid sinuses and the nasopharynx.

The morbidity related to primary intracranial tumors in humans is of considerable interest. The true incidence of primary intracranial neoplasms in our population cannot be determined from the mortality and surgical series data, which, according to Kurland et al.,[63] fail to provide adequate information. The most complete population survey of intracranial tumors available to date seems to be the report on a 10-year survey of the resident population of Rochester, Minnesota. From the Rochester data, Kurland[62] has estimated that, in a city of one million population, 142 new cases of intracranial neoplasms should be found each year, for both sexes combined: 77 of these would be primary tumors of the brain, 15 would be pituitary tumors, and 50 would be cases of intracranial metastases. For primary brain tumors, the incidence increases steadily with age.

In relation to neoplastic diseases, the incidence of primary intracranial neoplasms is relatively low, as it represents only 1.5 to 2 per cent of all primary neoplasms of the human body. The incidence of primary brain tumor increases steadily with age and rises sharply between the ages of 40 and 60, a period over which the average annual incidence doubles. The incidence appears to be slightly greater in males than in females. Tumors occur more frequently in the cerebrum than in any other part of the central nervous system. In children, the incidence is greater in the cerebellum and in the brain stem.

The mortality rates for all types of neoplasms of the nervous system in the United States and Canada reveal a remarkably even geographic distribution of such cases, as the rates range from 3 to 5 deaths per 100,000 population (Kurland et al.).[63] Considering that 45 to 50 per cent of the neoplasms of the nervous system are primary brain tumors, the mortality rates for primary brain tumors would average approximately 1.5 to 2.5 per 100,000 population. In Rochester, 1 per cent of all deaths which occurred over 10 years were due to primary intracranial tumors. The rates suggest that one of every 3 persons who develop a primary brain tumor might eventually die from that tumor.

I have endeavored to present here a comprehensive study of all pertinent factors related to the natural history and behavior of primary intracranial tumors. Perhaps this study would be incomplete without brief genetic considerations. The role that heredity may play in the causation of brain tumors has been studied and reviewed recently (1962) by Kurland, Myrianthopoulos and Lessell,[63] who have come to the conclusion that "for most types of brain tumors there is no clear cut evidence for or against a genetic mechanism." This is applicable to the gliomas in particular, the largest single group of brain tumors. As yet, there appears to be no definite evidence of difference in racial susceptibility.

EVALUATION OF METHODS OF DIAGNOSIS AND TUMOR LOCALIZATION

The therapeutic radiologist cannot judiciously use ionizing radiation in the treatment of primary intracranial neoplasms unless he has full knowledge of the localization and extent of the tumor to be irradiated in each individual case.

The advances made in neurologic diagnostic procedures in the last 20 years have been so considerable that the diagnosis of intracranial neoplasms can be made with increasing precision. Their exact location and actual size can be determined with a remarkable degree of accuracy. The relative advantages and limitations also of each method of investigation, either radiologic or nonradiologic, are better known and understood than ever before, so that the necessity for combining the use of two or more diagnostic procedures has become imperative in the diagnosis and localization of each lesion. Radiotherapists must be conversant with the degree of valid information which may be derived from each procedure and used for guidance in the planning of individual treatment.

Special radiologic x-ray examinations with contrast media provide radiation therapists with more adequate practical information than any other group of diagnostic procedures for the planning of treatment with ionizing radiation.

Pneumoencephalography and ventriculography with gas continue to allow the visualization of the ventricular system and the convolutional subarachnoid spaces better than by any other method of investigation. Brain tumors can be accurately diagnosed and localized by pneumograms in more than 90 per cent of the cases. Intraventricular, thalamic, occipital and posterior parasagittal tumors are usually best demonstrated by pneumogram. This also applies to tumors located in the mid-brain and in

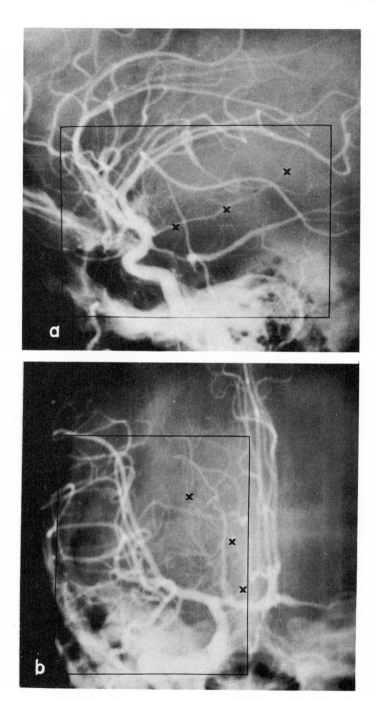

the suprasellar region. Infratentorial tumors occupying the posterior fossa like tumors of the 4th ventricle, cerebellum and brain-stem are ordinarily visualized more readily with pneumograms. In the cerebral hemispheres, pneumograms may show tumors when angiograms are negative or vice versa. In selected cases the use of dense contrast media for ventriculography may assist in demonstrating the location and size of tumors in the 3rd and 4th ventricles or in the brain stem, tumors which are difficult to demonstrate otherwise. Occasionally tomographic studies are made at the same time as ventriculography and may add to the accuracy of brain tumor localization.

Cerebral angiography has become an extremely useful method of radiological examination capable of establishing the presence of an intracranial tumor and its exact location by the extent and character of the modifications of the normal vascular pattern (Fig. 1a, b). Cerebral angiograms may also give some remarkable indications as to the probable histopathological type of tumor by demonstrating the blood circulation within the neoformed capillaries of the tumor itself. Meningiomas frequently have a characteristic angiographic pattern and they are by far the commonest intracranial tumors to have a double blood supply through the external carotid and the internal carotid or the vertebral artery. Glioblastomas often can be diagnosed by their vascular pattern which is nearly angiomatous in appearance in the late arterial, capillary and early venous phases, because of the large number of neo-formed capillaries containing blood with radio-opaque contrast media within the tumor itself. This is seen particularly well at the periphery of the glioblastoma, a very useful guide as to the size and extent of the tumor. Other tumors like the astrocytomas and the oligodendrogliomas ordinarily exhibit no special vascular pattern within the tumor itself and can be demonstrated by angiography merely by the displacement of blood vessels adjacent to the tumor. It is generally considered that 75 per cent of intracranial tumors can be demonstrated by angiography. It is possible to observe a practically normal angiogram in the presence of some intracranial tumors particularly in the case of intraventricular and brain stem tumors. Posterior fossa tumors may be demonstrated by a vertebral artery angiography, although its accuracy is not as good as carotid angiograms are for tumors located in the cerebral hemispheres.

Figure 1 a, On right lateral carotid angiogram, there is displacement of blood vessels by fair size tumor in right temporal lobe. The middle cerebral artery is displaced upward; the anterior choroidal is marked with three x. The posterior communicating and posterior cerebral arteries are displaced downward.

b, On antero-posterior right carotid angiogram, there is displacement upward and mesially of middle cerebral artery and most branches. Note particularly the extreme mesial position of the choroidal artery marked with three x.
Outline of suitable location and size of fields for radiation therapy were determined from angiographic study as shown by black rectangular demarcation on both a and b.

Gamma encephalography, the localization of intracranial neoplasms with radioactive isotopes, is another radiologic method which may assist in the determination of the size and exact location of human brain tumors. The accuracy of this method would appear to be reliable as yet in not more than 50 per cent of the cases. The best results have been reported in meningiomas and also in glioblastomas, that is in tumors with increased vascularization. Recently Raimondi[91] has reported that the tumor itself will pick up the circulating isotope in the blood stream and bring it into the cytoplasm of the neoplastic cells. Neoplastic astrocytes have an enhanced uptake.

Until recently there was virtually no accurate non-radiologic method of localization of intracranial neoplasm. Echo-encephalograms are now obtained with ultrasonic waves and in favorably situated tumors may accurately determine the size and location of intracranial lesions. Thermographic scan is another new method of localization of certain intracranial tumors; it is based upon the detection and recording of the infrared irradiation from abnormal blood vessels over them. The detection and accurate localization of intracranial tumors by this method has been reported recently by Goldberg, Heinz and Taveras.[41]

Electroencephalography is providing useful information regarding abnormal cerebral activity at the edges of a brain tumor, but, in general, it cannot be depended upon for guidance in the precise localization of tumors. In a small percentage of patients with supratentorial tumors, the electroencephalogram may even be normal. Infratentorial tumors involving the cerebellum or the brain stem are usually not detectable by electroencephalography, except in children.

Considering that the majority of primary intracranial tumors are irradiated postoperatively, the surgeons' observations recorded in the operative report should provide most valuable information concerning the identification, location and extent of the tumor.

Initial surgical management of the majority of primary intracranial neoplasms has the advantage of making tissue available for histopathological studies which permit the identification of the type of tumor and its classification. In several cases (10 to 12 per cent) in which craniotomy and surgical removal is not advisable, biopsy material adequate for pathologic studies and classification may be obtained by needle biopsy taken through twist drill holes made in the calvarium.

CLASSIFICATION AND PATHOLOGY OF INTRACRANIAL NEOPLASMS

There are approximately 30 different histopathologic types of primary intracranial neoplasms. These are quite distinct clinical and pathologic entities. Obviously some acceptable classification is required, if any critical comparative evaluation of the efficacy of treatment methods is to be made in relation with intracranial tumors. In a broad and general classification proposed by Bailey[8], the primary intracranial neoplasms have been grouped in accordance to certain resemblances in structure and behavior, as follow:

1) Encephalic tumors, including gliomas and glioneuromas.
2) Tumors of the covering cells of the nervous system, including meningeal tumors and sheath tumors.
3) Hypophyseal tumors, including adenomas and craniopharyngiomas.
4) Dysembryomas, including pinealomas and chordomas.
5) Vascular tumors.

The histopathology of tumors of the central nervous system is difficult and complex. This is particularly true for the gliomas, which represent approximately 50 per cent of all primary intracranial neoplasms. The pathological classification of the other intracranial neoplastic entities is not so complicated because they are more readily identified and their histopathologic characteristics are closely related to the structure of the tissue from which they have originated.

Tumors arising from neurones have not yet been identified and reported. This observation is also valid in the field of experimental brain tumors. In Zimmerman's experience[126], the only tumors induced in the cerebral cortex and basal ganglions were glial in origin.

The histopathological classification followed in our institution has been largely the one proposed by Bailey and Cushing[7]. The terminology used by pathologists in the classification of gliomas can be and often is very confusing. Unless one becomes familiar with the equivalent appellation given by pathologists to identical types of gliomas, it is virtually impossible to compare results of treatment, notwithstanding the variations in individual interpretation and classification. The necessity for such interpretation of terminology in the classification of primary intracranial gliomas has been recognized by neuropathologists to the extent that Zimmerman[123] and also Zulch[127] have prepared and published tables of synonyms or equivalent terminology. It has been suggested that the classification of gliomas be reviewed and simplified.

Intracranial gliomas are primary brain tumors arising from the glial cells of which three different types are generally recognized: the astrocytes, the oligodendrocytes and the ependymal cells. Gliomas arising from the astrocytic group of cells represent approximately three quarters of all primary intracranial gliomatous tumors. They give rise to tumors of variable degrees of differentiation and often bring the neuropathologist difficulties in differentiating the intermediate morphologic changes between the more malignant glioblastoma multiforme and the less malignant astrocytoma. In attempting to solve this classification problem, Ringertz[100], in 1950, has suggested a three-step grading of the astrocytic types of tumors, as follow: glioblastoma, intermediate type, astrocytoma. Kernohan *et al.*[55] has proposed to call them all astrocytomas, with a grading varying from I to IV to indicate the degree of differentiation of each tumor. Tumors originating from the oligodendroglial cells appear to be identified easily. Gliomas derived from the ependymal cells are relatively uncommon just like the oligodendrogliomas.

Zimmerman[124] has called attention to gliomas which are mixed tumors and contain portions of astrocytoma, oligodendroglioma, ependymoma or other types of glial neoplasms. He has also seen many mixed tumors in experimentally induced gliomas in animals. Furthermore he has reported that different strains of cells in a mixed glioma could be separated up in pure culture by the multiple transplant method, and eventually become pure astrocytomas or ependymomas.

Medulloblastomas are still classified with the gliomas by the majority of neuropathologists. However, there are conflicting opinions about their histogenesis. Some believe that such tumors more properly belong to the group of neuroblastomas and should be classified as such. Medulloblastomas represent approximately 10 per cent of all intracranial gliomas. They are notorious for their tendency to disseminate along the cerebrospinal axis in the subarachnoid spaces and also into the ventricular system. Cerebellar sarcomas and ependymoblastomas may at times be difficult to differentiate from medulloblastomas.

2
Radiobiologic Effects on the Central Nervous Tissues and Tumors

ANY RADIATION THERAPIST, who accepts the responsibility of treating primary intracranial neoplasms or any other type of lesion of the central nervous system, should be fully conversant with the immediate and late biological effects of ionizing radiation on nervous tissue and other intracranial structures, as well as on tumors of a variety of histopathologic types. It is imperative for one to be familiar with the radiation tolerance of the central nervous system tissues in order to avoid exceeding, in clinical radiation therapy, the amounts of radiation which can be administered safely over a certain period of time. Yet, the doses delivered must be adequate enough to accomplish the biologic effects desired, without inducing undue reaction at any time.

It is difficult to assess fully the effect of irradiation in the treatment of neoplasms of the central nervous system. Obviously, it is impossible to irradiate an intracranial tumor without, at the same time, irradiating equally the intervening or adjacent nervous tissues. The radiobiologic tolerance of the latter tissues may vary considerably and be conditioned by their relatively normal or diseased state at the onset of treatment.

After the incidental exposure of brain tissue contiguous to a tumor treated with ionizing radiation, the tissue changes, either gross or microscopic, which are interpreted as postradiation cerebral reactions are not pathognomonic. Identical changes are commonly observed in the brain of patients whose tumor has never been irradiated. In the latter instance the brain damage is attributed to increased intracranial pressure or to impaired cerebral blood circulation or to some other cause which may be related with the tumor alone. Postradiation effects on the primary brain tumor itself are also difficult to evaluate, considering that most of the gross and histopathologic changes observed within the irradiated tumors may be seen in non-irradiated tumors as well.

It has been stated that in man the normal nervous tissue is highly radioresistant. In fact, any degree of radiation effect may develop in the normal

29

brain and range from the unidentifiable to gross degenerative changes. The radiobiologic effects vary mostly in relation to the total dose and the manner in which radiation is administered, either in a single exposure or in divided doses protracted over different periods of time. The gross and microscopic changes seen in in the human brain adjacent to a primary tumor which has been irradiated are variable; often, these cannot be differentiated from the tissue changes which can be attributed to the tumor solely or to radiation alone.

The influence of local irradiation on the physiological and functional processes of the normal central nervous system is far from easy to determine and little is known about this. In animals, many investigators have reported that the functional state of the central nervous system is highly sensitive to ionizing radiation and may respond to doses as low as 10 rads, once the animals are adequately conditioned. In humans with brain tumors, irradiation must add to the existing profound disturbances of the physiological and functional processes in the brain itself primarily and, by repercussion, beyond the immediate cerebral zone. There is a great deal to be discovered by investigation of that aspect of radiobiology in humans.

ANALYSIS OF EXPERIMENTAL DATA IN ANIMALS

Considerable experimental evidence is available regarding the postradiation effects on animal normal nervous tissue, but its interpretation often requires a certain degree of circumspection. In that respect, Dyke and Davidoff[30] reviewed the literature up to 1939 and found the results difficult to evaluate for comparative purposes. Later, we[13] have summarized some of the experimental studies which were conducted on animals from 1938 to 1958 and, in our opinion, have contributed observations applicable to radiation therapy.

Contrast Between Experimental and Clinical Use of Radiation

In nearly every experiment the tissue changes noted have resulted from the administration of single incident doses varying from 1000 to 5000 r. Such changes in animal normal nervous tissue cannot be compared directly with the postradiation changes which might develop in man following radiation therapy of intracranial neoplasms, because the conditions of irradiation are far from being identical. Prior to irradiation, the animal brains were presumably normal, whereas most of the human brains affected with a tumor are already diseased to some degree. Furthermore, the single doses used in animal experiments have been far in excess of the dosage applied in the treatment of brain tumors in man. Indeed, single doses varying from 1000 to 5000 r must produce in the central nervous system of animals postradiation tissue changes different from those which may develop in the human brain following the administration of proportional total doses but administered in multiple fractions over a period of 30 to 50 days. Nevertheless some experimental observations have brought out certain radiobiologic facts which should be retained.

Experimental Radiation Effects Resembling Brain Tissue Reactions in Humans

Following animal experiments in which the investigators have employed conventional x-ray therapy apparatus at 200 kv., or the so-called orthovoltage, and have used single large doses of X-radiation the subsequent observations appear to be significant. Davidoff, Dyke, Elsberg and Tarlov[26] irradiated (1000 to 5000 r) the brain of monkeys directly through an open wound and later observed severe degeneration involving both nervous and glial cells; they found relatively slight changes in the blood vessels, and we presume that this was due to the relatively short time elapsed between irradiation and autopsy.

Reynolds[95] demonstrated that, in the brains of dogs, myelin is rather sensitive to X-radiation and that myelin damage gives the normal brain more radiosensitivity than expected; he also pointed out that myelin degeneration may be a late manifestation and take as long as one year to become demonstrable in experimental animals.

Dorothy S. Russell, C.W. Wilson and Katherine Tensley[102] described experimenal radionecrosis induced in the brains of rabbits by external irradiation, following single surface doses varying from 1625 to 2850 r. The rabbits were sacrificed at various times up to 234 days or more. A latent period up to 100 days was noted in the rabbits which had received 2850 r. The initial histologic changes consisted of minute foci of hemorrhage and necrosis. The lesions, once established, extended rapidly and widely to the non-irradiated portions of the brain. In the late stages, gliosis with progressive degeneration and sclerosis of the adjacent blood vessels was noted. Neurones were only affected secondarily in spots.

Clements and Holst[20] used trypan blue to demonstrate the pathologic changes in the neurones, neuroglia and blood brain barrier following single exposures of 1500 to 6000 r in monkeys. The degree of blue staining appeared to be directly proportional to the dose, since it was quite marked and constant with the higher doses. Astrocytic degeneration and severe neuronal damage were observed side by side. They noted that the hypothalamus, optic thalamus and brain stem were most often colored and therefore more radiosensitive.

Experimental investigation of the effects on the brain of high energy X-radiation from the 23 mev. betatron was reported by Arnold, Bailey and Laughlin[4]. They used adult monkeys and administered single exposures ranging from 1500 to 14000 r, and the animals were killed at various intervals up to 24 months. In the relatively low dose range of 1500 to 3000 r, they observed immediate acute changes with mild degrees of degeneration, and late radionecrosis 12 to 24 months after exposure. They concluded that high energy X-radiation induced in the brain of the monkey effects which are largely direct rather than secondary to vascular changes and that the central nervous system is more radioresponsive than is generally believed. Arnold, Bailey and Harvey[2] also applied the high energy X-radiation of the 23 mev. betatron to the temporal lobes and brain stem of monkeys. Single doses of 3000 r induced delayed radionecrosis of the brain stem with marked damage in the fiber tracts. They also reported that the hypothalamus appeared to be very sensitive to high energy radiation at the dose level of 3000 r.

Phases in Development of Brain Damage Induced by Single Massive Doses

The experimental work briefly reviewed above has clearly revealed that single massive doses of ionizing radiation are capable of inducing severe postradiation damage in the normal central nervous tissues of animals. In every experiment there was a latent period between irradiation and initial evidence of radiobiologic effects. The length of the latent period was inversely proportional to the magnitude of the dose administered, the higher the dose, the shorter the latent period.

In the acute and relatively immediate postradiation reactions, the degree of severity and the extent of the lesions appeared to be directly proportional to the dose-intensity. Once established the lesions could extend to the non-irradiated portions of the brain. These initial effects have apparently resulted from direct damage to the glial cells and from degenerative changes associated with acute vascular reactions involving the capillaries in particular, whereas neuronal damage seemed to be less marked and often undetectable.

The late postradiation effects on the other hand would consist of slow and progressing degenerative changes secondary to lesions of the larger blood vessels, arterioles and arteries, and the radiation damage eventually resulted in brain necrosis. Myelin is rather sensitive to X-radiation and it seems that brain damage follows closely the demyelinization of nerve tracts. The white matter would appear to be more vulnerable than the gray matter except in the mid-brain and brain stem where both seem to be equally vulnerable.

EFFECTS OF IRRADIATION OF NORMAL BRAIN TISSUE IN HUMANS

The true effects of ionizing radiation on the normal human brain and the rest of the intracranial content cannot be determined accurately by studying the tissue reactions which may be observed in patients irradiated for primary intracranial neoplasms. The main reason is that, when a patient is subjected to radiation therapy for an intracranial neoplasm, the brain and adjacent tissues are no longer in their normal state but are diseased in some degree.

Radiation Tolerance Observed After Treatment of Extracranial Lesions

In humans, the radiation tolerance of the normal brain and other intracranial structures can be studied with strict scientific objectivity only from patients whose intracranial content was casually exposed to radiation therapy. This has occurred in patients who presumably had perfectly normal brains at the time that some zone of their brain was irradiated since it happened to be located directly beneath an extracranial lesion treated with ionizing radiation. Lampe[65] has noted that, with few exceptions, the non-nervous tissue lesions treated, "when parts of the central nervous system have been included in the irradiated zone, have been neoplastic lesions requiring the therapeutic administration of relatively large radiation doses". Several authors have reported damage to the brain and other intracranial structures following irradiation of malignant tumors of the scalp.

Sizable single doses of ionizing radiation have been administered in the treatment of extracranial lesions. The radiation tolerance of the underlying normal human brain tissue should be commensurate with that of the normal animal brain tissue investigated under similar conditions of exposure to radiation. The nervous tissue reactions should be more or less identical in both instances.

In a case reported by Pennybacker and Russell[87] the patient developed brain necrosis beneath the site of a rodent ulcer 9 months after a single dose of 2300 r (in air) and the necrosis was proved by microscopic studies after surgical removal of the cerebral lesion. The x-ray treatment had been administered at 230 kv. to a circular field of 7 cm. in diameter. Lowenberg-Scharenberg and Bassett[70] also reported a case of brain necrosis following a single massive dose of 3000 r (air) for a cancer of the skin located over the right parietal area. A field 5 x 6 cm. was exposed to unfiltered X-radiation generated at 110 and 130 kv. The latent period was longer than in the first case as the clinical symptoms of brain damage developed almost 42 instead of 9 months after irradiation.

The gross and microscopic findings observed in the 2 cases of brain necrosis reported above have developed after single massive doses of X-radiation to normal human brains. Such observations suggest that single tissue doses in the range of 2400 to 3000 r or more might exceed the radiation tolerance of the normal brain in man. In animal experiments, single doses of comparable magnitude (2400 r) have been reported to exceed the radiation tolerance of normal brain and single tissue doses of 30003 r have invariably induced brain necrosis.

Postirradiation Brain Necrosis Simulating Gliomas

Brain necrosis following the incidental irradiation of a zone of the normal central nervous tissue in the treatment of an extracranial lesion may simulate a glioma. The clinical picture presented by the patient is such that all symptoms and objective findings suggest an intracranial space-occupying lesion. In a case reported by Lowenberg-Scharenberg and Bassett[70], the patient was treated for a basal cell carcinoma located over the left temple. This lesion of the scalp received a total dose of 6000 r (measured in air) over a period of 12 days at 150 kv., the field covering an area of approximately 24 square centimeters. A second course of roentgen therapy was administered 22 months after the first for a presumptive recurrence and the same area was exposed to an additional dose of 3600 r at the rate of 150 r daily with 180 kv. radiation. She showed evidence of an intracranial space-occupying lesion 49 months after the second course of irradiation and 71 months after the first. At operation, the lesion grossly resembled a glioma. Microscopically it showed necrotic substance and was diagnosed amyloid degeneration of the brain secondary to irradiation of the scalp neoplastic lesion.

A similar case of brain necrosis, in which the diagnosis of glioma of the astrocytic type was made initially, was reported by Dugger, Stratford and Bouchard.[29] The patient had received at another hospital a dose of 4800 r (air dose) at 150 kv. over a period of 10 days to an area measuring 5 cm. in diameter. We later estimated the surface dose at 5500 r and the depth doses at 4000 r at 2.5 cm. and 2750 r at 5 cm. in the brain tissue of the temporal lobe. Following this treatment the carcinoma involving the skin over the temporal region regressed and the lesion healed. Approximately 26 months after irradiation, he developed clinical and neuroradiologic evidence of a space-occupying lesion in the temporal horn and lateral ventricle, immediately beneath the extracranial area which was irradiated. At operation the lesion looked like a glioma and on the frozen sections the histologic diagnosis of astrocytoma was made (Fig. 2a, b). Postoperative roentgen therapy was initiated but was soon discontinued when the tumor dose had reached 2340 r in 32 days and the clinical and microscopic correlation of all the evidence available clearly established that this was a case of localized brain necrosis which had developed in the normal brain tissue located beneath a heavily irradiated carcinoma of the scalp. This patient recovered and enjoyed a relatively good survival. He had minimal residual signs but persistent nominal aphasia.

Many years after the publication of the latter case report, in effect 9 years after craniotomy and extirpation of the postradiation brain lesion, the patient died suddenly from coronary thrombosis associated with generalized arteriosclerosis. At autopsy, the intracranial changes were confined

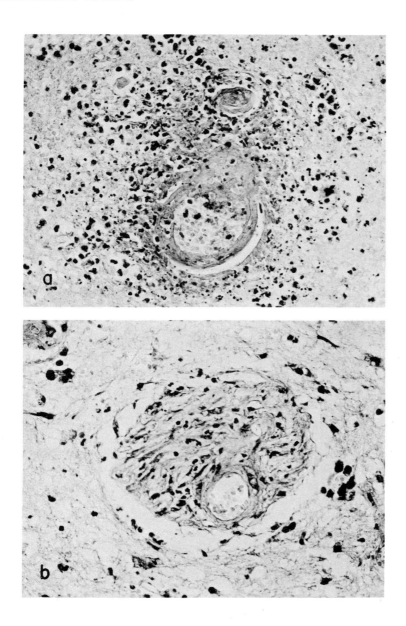

Figure 2 a, Thickening and recent necrosis of vessel wall in left temporal lobe; necrosis and cellular reaction in surrounding brain. Hematoxylin and van Giesen stain, x 280. Case of radiation necrosis simulating astrocytoma.

b, Fibrous proliferation of adventitia of an intracerebral vessel; gliosis of surrounding brain. Hematoxylin and van Giesen x 280.

to the affected temporal lobe, where they consisted of localized gliosis and atrophy of the white matter which was largely destroyed at the site of the previously extirpated lesion of radiation necrosis. There was a lesser degree of cortical damage with moderate degeneration of the neurones. A striking feature was the minimal changes observed in the blood vessels. No trace was found of the previous presumptive astrocytoma.

Normal Brain Tolerance to Radiation Exceeded by Large Doses and Repeated Courses

The last two reports are most significant. They bring highly informative radiobiologic observations concerning radiation effects and manifestations which are presumably uncommon in relation with the tolerance of the normal central nervous tissue in humans, and for which there is no parallel experimental evidence. Both cases illustrate the danger of irradiating normal human brain with total doses which are relatively large when administered in single or in divided exposures over short periods of time. The radiation tolerance of normal brain tissue may be more easily exceeded when the volume of tissue irradiated with such large doses surpasses 50 to 75 cc., because the amount of radiation absorbed is then high.

The first report also suggests that the repetition of courses of irradiation may be a decisive factor in producing brain necrosis in consideration of cumulative effects, particularly when the initial course administered had been intensive. The air dose levels which reached 6000 r in 12 days initially and 3600 r in 24 days subsequently in a repeat exposure obviously were not well tolerated by the brain and seemed to have exceeded the radiation tolerance of normal human nervous tissue.

The length of latent periods before brain necrosis will manifest itself may vary considerably. The initial acute reaction, which can occur after massive single doses or following intensive irradiation in divided doses, seemed to cause no detectable symptoms in the above cases of late necrosis of normal brain tissue as clinically such reaction passed unnoticed. The microscopic changes observed were identified as those of late postradiation injury in both cases, but not at first in our own case in which the picture resembled and simulated an astrocytoma presumably because of the reaction of the astrocytes.

POSTRADIATION EFFECTS ON CEREBRAL AND OTHER INTRACRANIAL TISSUES INVOLVED IN THE TREATMENT OF MALIGNANT INTRACRANIAL NEOPLASMS

Reduced Radiation Tolerance of Nervous Tissue Adjacent to Brain Tumors

The evaluation of postradiation changes in the human brain following the treatment of intracranial tumors with large doses of ionizing radiation is a judicious task. One has to try and differentiate between morphologic changes which are practically identical, whether they have been induced by generalized increased intracranial pressure or by the local tumor growth or possibly by radiation. The fact that the brain adjacent to a tumor is already diseased to some degree, in part or in toto, at the onset of irradiation must render the brain tissue more vulnerable to large doses of radiation than if it were normal to begin with. In other words, in the presence of a primary intracranial neoplasm the radiation tolerance of the surrounding central nervous tissue must be diminished by comparison with that of the normal human brain.

There should be no denial of the accumulated evidence which demonstrates that postradiation encephalitis and localized brain necrosis may develop subsequently to the irradiation of an intracranial neoplasm. However, the incidence of such complications seems to be relatively uncommon and should remain low. Postradiation brain damage is a late complication which is avoidable in the treatment of patients affected with intracranial neoplasms. The potential risk that such complication might occur should not deprive a patient of the opportunity of a good recovery and long survival that adequate radiation therapy may provide. To prevent adverse and unnecessary complications, it is imperative to take advantage of the experience provided from the studies of the normal brain tissue tolerance to irradiation in man primarily and to some extent in experimental animals. Equally important is the study of the many reports of postradiation brain damage subsequent to irradiation of malignant intracranial neoplasms. One must endeavor to determine and understand every factor which may contribute to the induction of such complications.

Reports on Postradiation Brain Necrosis

Wachowski and Cheneault[116] published their experience with 6 patients, who were treated for brain tumors and received postoperative tumor doses varying between 6100 and 8800 r in 85 to 100 days, and later developed evidence of intracranial degenerative effects. The tissue changes described were affecting all the cellular elements. There was almost complete disintegration of the nerve cells of the cerebral cortex. The neuroglial cells were swollen and contained fat in their cytoplasm. Microglia had increased in number. The capillaries were showing an excessive amount of fat lying in the endothelial or adventitial cells, but the large blood vessels were in a good state of preservation. The authors expressed their belief that such changes would not be due solely to the presence of neoplasms nor to increased intracranial pressure but represented radiation effects.

Pennybacker and Dorothy Russell[87] described the clinical and pathologic features of postradiation brain necrosis that they observed in 4 patients previously irradiated for intracranial tumors. The latent period between radiation therapy and the onset of clinical signs extended from 10 months to 5 years. In all 4 cases the cerebral lesions consisted of extensive sub-cortical necrosis which was apparent in practically every portion of the brain but was maximal in the field which had received the most irradiation. In their opinion the critical level of blood vessel changes is reached many months or years after irradiation so that gradual ischemia results in a slow onset of the clinical and neurohistologic changes, whereas vascular throm-bosis would bring on an acute onset.

Arnold, Bailey and Harvey[2] have reported delayed necrosis of the brain stem and hypothalamus in 2 patients one year or more following the treat-ment of brain stem gliomas, having used tumor doses of 4500 r of 400 Kv x-rays in 30 days.

Lampe and MacIntyre[64] have reported their experience in relation to late radiation damage of the brain in cases of medulloblastoma of the cerebellum. Of 26 patients, 7 survived beyond 5 years. Brain damage has occurred in 4 of the 7 survivors. Two were perfectly normal for approxi-mately 12 and 13 years after irradiation. The seventh patient presented questionable signs of radiation damage 15 years after treatment. In 1950, Lampe[65] altered his method of irradiation to a fractional technique pro-tracted over 55 to 65 days using an estimated dose of 5000 to 6000 r. At the time of a subsequent report (1957) he had treated 7 patients who could be observed for 3 years or longer. Four of the 7 had already survived from 3 to 6 years and all 4 were in good health.

The only identified case of postradiation brain necrosis in our own series showed extensive bilateral necrosis of the occipital lobes, with evi-dence of residual or recurrent tumor at the site of the primary lesion in the right cerebellum. This resulted from 2 intensive courses of roentgen ther-apy administered for a perithelial sarcoma (Fig. 3 a, b) located in the right cerebellar lobe. In the first course of irradiation, the patient (5½ years old) received postoperatively a tumor dose of 6500 r in 38 days to the entire intracranial content, and 2000 r in 18 days to the spinal axis as the diagnosis of medulloblastoma was considered just as probable as that of sarcoma. Subsequently she was symptom-free for nearly 3 years. She then presented with signs of recurrence and it was agreed that she should be treated again with radiation. The tumor-bearing area received a further dose of 5300 rads over a period of 60 days. She died almost 3 years after the second course of roentgen therapy, altogether 70 months after the initial irradia-tion. Her vision deteriorated gradually during the last 18 months and she was completely blind when she died.

The diagnosis of postradiation brain necrosis was made in our case during the terminal phase and it was confirmed by post-mortem exami-nation. Both cerebral hemispheres showed well defined zones of brain necrosis through the occipital lobes (Fig. 4) and this location of brain damage was conforming to distribution of the opposing lateral beams of X-radiation used in the treatment of this case of intracranial sarcoma. The

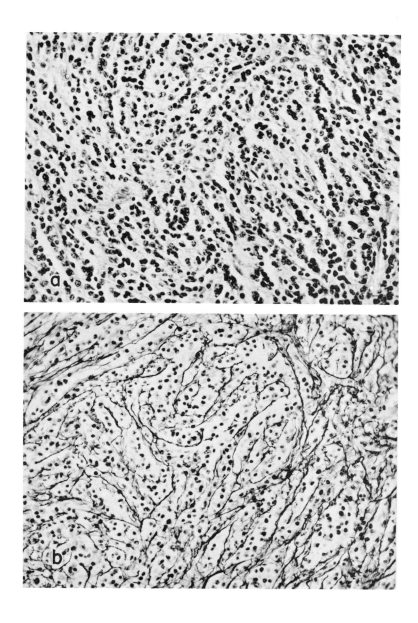

Figure 3 a Cerebellar tumor in 5½ year old child. Hematoxylin, phloxine, saffran stain, x 280

b, Same tumor as Fig. 4, Laidlaws stain showing abundant reticulin network. x 280

histologic changes were similar to the late tissue reactions described by most observers, and they consisted of widespread degenerative changes most striking near the blood vessels and in their lumen (Fig 5 a, b). Extensive gliosis was observed near the degenerated area. The damage involved both the grey and the white matter, but was more marked in the

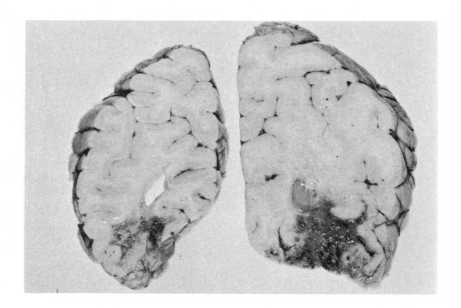

Figure 4, Bilateral occipital lobe necrosis, nearly 7 years after irradiation of patient whose cerebellar tumor is depicted in Figs 3 a and 3 b. (see case report)

white substance, and this extended beyond the tissue directly exposed to radiation into the temporal lobes. Recurrent or residual sarcoma was found in right cerebellum.

Several observers have noted that postradiation damage was particularly severe in the zones which had received the most irradiation, as we found in our case. In some cases the reaction was extending to practically every other portion of the brain. Reynolds[95] was able to demonstrate myelin damage in the uninvaded hemisphere of human brains treated with radiation therapy for intracranial malignant neoplasm.

Clinical Pattern in Brain Necrosis and Differential Diagnosis

A clinical pattern appears to be more or less identical and constant in all patients who have developed postradiation brain necrosis. Following

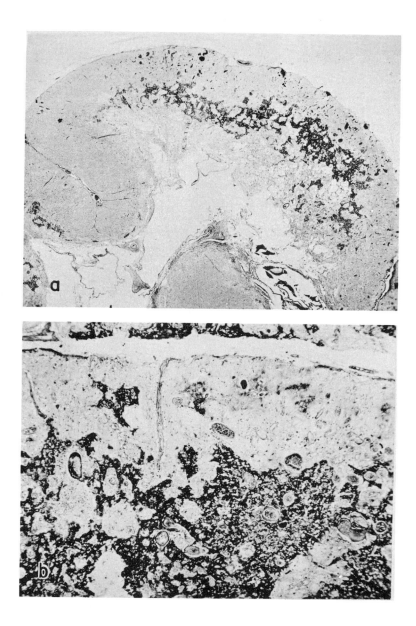

Figure 5 a, Postirradiation brain necrosis in occipital lobe. Cavitation of white matter with lesser involvement of overlying cortex. Phosphotungstic acid hematoxylin stain, x 8. Same case as Fig. 4.

   b, Numerous thick-walled blood vessels and dark-staining proteinaceous coagulum in cortex. Phosphotungstic acid hematoxylin, x 38. Same case as Fig. 4.

treatment, a period of improvement and even total recovery usually happens and this condition may persist for 1 to 5 years or longer. Sudden or gradual deterioration of the patient's clinical condition may develop without signs of increased intracranial pressure, *i.e.* without papilledema or increased tension at a level of the osteoplastic flap. Neurologic signs are present but vary in relation to the cerebral territory directly damaged by radiation. Such clinical pattern has been considered by most observers as evidence of postradiation damage of the central nervous tissue. The overall picture must be differentiated from deterioration of clinical condition associated with evidence of tumor reactivation or progression, thrombosis or hemorrhage, abscess or other inflammatory process.

The majority of immediate complications or late sequelae are attributable to the tumor itself rather than to the use of radiation, alone or in combination with surgery, in the course of treatment. Too often, residual clinical manifestations which have not regressed following treatment are also considered as sequelae of the treatment applied, especially when radiation has been used. Reactivation of tumor and concomitant deterioration of a patient's condition is often attributed unduly to postradiation damage.

Excessive Doses or Repeated Courses Related to Postirradiation Brain Necrosis

In reviewing reports of proven cases of postradiation necrosis observed at various sites of the central nervous system in humans following radiation therapy of primary intracranial tumors, one is impressed with the fact that such complications appear to have developed mostly under two sets of circumstances, either of which may have been sufficient to play a paramount role in inducing such complication. The first hazard seems to be the administration of large tumor doses, which may be excessive when delivered over a relatively short period of time (3000 to 5000 rads in 2 to 3 weeks) or even when protracted over longer periods of time if the doses are very high. The second hazard and often the most common appears to be the repetition of series of treatment over a period of 1 year or even much longer, in which moderate to large doses of ionizing radiation are directed to the same regions of the central nervous system during each course of treatment with radiation.

We have accumulated considerable evidence that *postradiation injury of the brain can be avoided by fractionation and protraction of radiation doses in a single continuous series.* The importance of protraction and fractionation of dose in the treatment by irradiation of intracranial neoplasms has been demonstrated by the absence of immediate histopathologic changes in the peritumoral neurones, glial cells, blood vessels and meninges. In cases in which the dose has been fractionated within the range of accepted tissue doses (approximately 5000 rads over periods varying from 30 to 50 days), there were no appreciable postradiation tissue changes observed beyond the tumor-bearing area, either immediately or even months to years later. Such observations were made repeatedly in the several cases whose autopsy I attended, and also in a number of post-mortem microscopic studies recorded by our neuropathologists. In more than 30 of the patients who were irradiated postoperatively and were subsequently re-operated upon for tumor recurrence, Cone and Elvidge[22] observed no gross evidence of degenerative changes other than those usu-ally found as results of their tumor alone.

Radiation Tolerance of Human Brain Tissue

From the above considerations it is quite clear that adequate irradiation of primary intracranial neoplasms can be accomplished without inducing postradiation injury in the adjacent brain tissue and other intracranial structures. It is also undisputable that late postradiation necrosis may de-velop in the peritumoral brain tissue in some of the cases. Such dual and diametrically different potential postradiation effects raise the question of the determination of the dose range that the brain might tolerate and cannot be exceeded without risking immediate or late undue postradiation reactions. Because of variation in technique, in volume irradiated, in the condition of the vascular system and because perhaps of other factors which may complicate the situation, Lampe[65] expressed the opinion that the precise radiation tolerance limits of the central nervous system are not clearly known and that a definitive radiation tolerance dose for clinical purposes may never be known.

And yet, several workers have attempted to determine dose levels which might be used safely in the treatment of primary intracranial neoplasms. Most of the radiation tolerance doses suggested have been expressed in terms of definite time periods for the administration of radiation therapy, since it is recognized that dose and time are the basic factors combining to determine the true magnitude of irradiation intensity and of all radio-biologic effects. Boden[12] has emphasized the importance of a third major factor in relation to the radiation tolerance of the central nervous tissue. This factor is the magnitude of the volume of tissue exposed to radiation. He has demonstrated that the dose tolerance of brain tissue is inversely proportional with the volume of tissue subjected to irradiation: the smaller the volume the greater the tolerance to radiation, and the larger the volume the lesser the tolerance.

Radiation Tolerance Curves for Brain

The limits of radiation tolerance of brain tissue have been studied by several investigators who have suggested levels of irradiation intensity that could be considered safe. Boden gave an upper limit of 3500 r depth dose in 17 days when large field techniques were used and 4500 r in 17 days with small field techniques. Effectively, Boden[11] was first (1948) to publish radiation tolerance curves applicable to the brain stem and the rest of the human brain. These curves emerged from a careful scrutiny of the dosimetry in 10 cases of radiation myelitis which developed in the cervical spinal cord following irradiation for head and neck neoplasms. Later, Boden[12] also reported brain stem damage in 7 patients who developed symptoms of pontine degeneration 11 to 20 months after radiation therapy for lesions near the base of the skull.

From Boden's tolerance curves, dosage biologically equivalent can be obtained readily in relation to the highest dose that the brain stem and the rest of the brain may tolerate over certain periods of time and in consideration also of the volume of brain tissue exposed to radiation. Boden used Strandquist's curves for skin necrosis and, on the basis of the depth doses that the brain and cord could tolerate in 17 days (3500 to 4500 r), he arrived at the following biological equivalents for the central nervous tissue: 3650 to 4700 r in 21 days, 3900 to 5000 r in 28 days, 4100 to 5300 r in 35 days, 4300 to 5500 r in 42 days, 4500 to 5800 r in 49 days, and 4700 to 6100 r in 56 days. McWhirter and Dott[77] (1955) have stated that 5500 r tumor dose in 4 weeks is at the upper limit of brain tolerance, but they also indicated that it is desirable not to exceed 5000 r over the same period of time.

Lindgren[68] published time-dose relationship curves in respect to the incidence of radionecrosis in the human brain. His curves were based upon a total of 17 cases (13 from the literature and 4 from his own files) in which necrosis involved brain tissue that was considered free of tumor. He only accepted cases with complete data of dosimetry and histologic proof of cerebral injury. All patients had been irradiated in a single series, with fractionated doses in 15 of the 17 cases. Treatment covered a period of 0 to 105 days: 2 patients had received single doses, 3 had been treated within 10 days, whereas the others had been irradiated over periods ranging from 17 to 38 days and from 84 to 105 days. Using all the data available, Lindgren drew up a modified Strandquist's diagram (Chart 1) showing 2 logarithmic curves: (a) the upper line corresponds to the maximum dosage level above which the risk of cerebral necrosis is considerable; (b) the lower line shows the lowest level of dosage at which brain necrosis has been induced. The dose given is that received in the centre of the irradiated region. Of the 17 cases used by Lindgren in the making of his diagram of brain tolerance to irradiation, 10 lie above the line of maximum tolerance and 7 lie between the lines of maximum and minimum tolerance.

Lindgren has compared his dose level curves with the ones published by Boden (1950) and by Zeman (1950) and he has observed that the limits of brain tolerance to radiation, that each of them has shown individually,

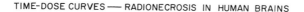

TIME-DOSE CURVES — RADIONECROSIS IN HUMAN BRAINS

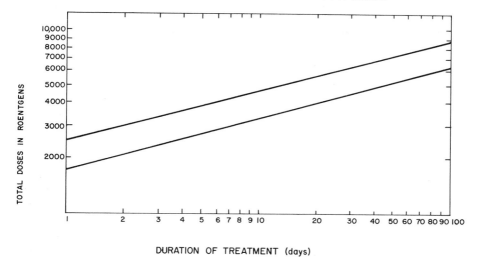

DURATION OF TREATMENT (days)

CHART I

Time-Dose Curves Made By Lindgren In Relation To Radionecrosis In Human Brains

lie below the upper limits obtained in his investigation, and therefore lie within the dosage range where the risk of necrosis is less pronounced. Furthermore, Lindgren has plotted the focal doses received by 5 of his patients still living in comfort 4 to 10 years after irradiation of brain tumors, and in 4 of the 5 the dose levels were lying on or below the lowest level producing necrosis whereas the dose in the remaining case was between the lines of minimum and maximum tolerance.

The time-dose relationship curves (Chart 1) for radionecrosis in human brains that Lindgren has calculated from collective precise data are the result of a considerable endeavor to assess the radiosensitivity of human brain tissue. These curves could serve as a safety guide in the management of any patient whose brain will be irradiated for an intracranial neoplasm or perhaps for some extracranial lesion. The use of Lindgren's curves might prevent one from exceeding the safe limits of exposure to ionizing radiation at both the high and low levels of brain tolerance. In Lindgren's opinion, of the two curves of his modified Strandquizt's diagram the lower is the more important because it indicates the lowest dosage level capable of producing cerebral necrosis in patients.

The dose-time range that we have considered and are still considering within the limits of brain tolerance in the irradiation of primary intracranial tumors consists of 5000 to 6000 rads tumor dose, administered over a period of approximately 50 days with a quality of radiation corresponding to that produced by kilovoltage x-ray apparatus.

It is generally agreed that the relative biological effects of high energy radiation are less intense than those of the lower energy level corresponding to kilovoltage. This difference in tissue reaction should be compensated by increasing tumor doses by 20 per cent when using Co^{60} gamma radiation or 4 Mev X-radiation. However we never exceed total tumor doses of 6500 rads over 50 days.

The tumor doses just mentioned are in agreement with Boden's upper limits of brain tolerance to radiation and fall below the upper and lower limits in Lindgren's curves. In view of our long-standing experience with irradiation of the brain surrounding primary cerebral gliomas and with exposure at the same time of the other intracranial structures, our long-term results strongly suggest that the time-dose relation used in the treatment of our patients probably represents an optimum range of tissue tolerance for the brain and the entire intracranial content. We sincerely believe that this statement will be adequately supported by the subsequent presentation of our long-term results.

In the case of late postradiation brain necrosis reported above with respect to one of our own patients, the tissue changes were observed beyond the site of the primary cerebellar sarcoma. The brain damage, which was found in both occipital lobes and extended into the temporal lobes, can be related to the following factors: (1) high intensity of irradiation (6500 rads in 38 days) which had exceeded the upper limits of brain tolerance in the first course alone; the period of time during which treatment was given was too short in view of the magnitude of dose and the volume of tissue exposed to such intensive irradiation; (2) the repetition of a sizable tumor dose (5300 rads in 60 days) to the posterior intracranial content; (3) the relative radioresistance of the primary tumor, which recurred almost 3 years after surgical extirpation and postoperative irradiation, was responsible for risking an additional series of treatment which did not prevent residual tumor from being found in the primary site at autopsy.

Lindgren reported that necrosis was found in the occipital lobes of 4 patients who had been irradiated for primary tumors involving the cerebellum: in 3 cases of medulloblastoma and in 1 case of malignant ependymoma. Two of these patients had received more than one course of radiation therapy. The other 2 were treated in single courses of irradiation, with protracted doses which aggregated to tumor doses of high intensity exceeding in 1 case the upper limit of tolerance (7500 r in 31 days) and in the other (5300 r in 34 days) surpassed the minimal limit of radiation tolerance of brain tissue.

Advantages of Megavoltage over Kilovoltage Radiation

The potential postradiation damage to normal brain, in the opinion of Jones [49], may be minimized by using high energy radiation. Amongst other advantages, megavoltage seems to be tolerated better than kilovoltage radiation, an important factor when one considers that the doses required in attempting to cure a brain tumor are often above the tolerance to kilovoltage radiation of the adjacent brain tissue. On the other hand, Arnold, Bailey, Harvey and Haas[3] have made histopathologic studies on cases of glioblastoma treated with megavoltage radiation, and their studies at operation or autopsy have revealed more intense changes than usually observed following kilovoltage x-ray therapy. These findings in our opinion would suggest that a greater degree of caution is indicated when using megavoltage if postradiation brain injury is to be avoided. Clinically their results of treatment of glioblastoma were apparently superior to those generally obtained with kilovoltage, but these were early observations. In the treatment of those patients with 23.0 mev. x-rays, Arnold et al.[3] used tumor doses varying from 5500 to 6500 rads in 17 to 30 days, up to 7500 rads in 26 to 30 days, a dose range which in the light of existing radiation tolerance curves would appear to be hazardous in regard to potential late brain necrosis.

In order to induce with megavoltage radiation relative biological effects of practically the same degree of intensity as those induced by kilovoltage radiation, a 25 per cent dose increase is suggested by Mitchell[79] for treatment with high energy radiation in the 20 to 30 mev. energy range. In making such tumor dose adjustments, the therapeutic radiologist must keep in mind that the lesser local reactions associated with the use of megavoltage have removed an obvious safeguard against the temptation of accumulating larger depth doses in a shorter time. One must be particularly cautious not to exceed the tolerance dose of the brain tissue adjacent to intracranial neoplasms under treatment. In terms of radiation tolerance of the central nervous system in humans, the words of wisdom written by Lampe[65] should be kept in mind: "Past experience does offer some rough guideline beyond which one may venture only at the risk of courting disaster".

Potential Incidental Radiation Effects on Pituitary Gland and Eyes

The possibility of postradiation damage to the pituitary gland in the treatment of intracranial neoplasms not arising from the gland itself must be considered. The hypophysis and its stalk are often damaged indirectly by an intracranial neoplasm causing erosion and enlargement of the sella turcica together with compression of the gland within the sella. In such cases the pituitary gland is no longer normal and may be more vulnerable to irradiation, when it happens to lie in the path of one or more beams of ionizing radiation directed primarily to a malignant intracranial tumor. Under the circumstances radiation injury may occur, but it must be rare within the range of tumor doses to which the pituitary may be exposed when the irradiated tumors are located in proximity to the sella turcica.

The normal pituitary gland can tolerate radiation well, within the range of therapeutic doses used in the treatment of intracranial neoplasms. Brain tolerance doses would have to be exceeded considerably for damage to be induced in the pituitary as result of irradiation of a brain tumor. It has been suggested that doses as high as 25,000 to 30,000 rads may be required to destroy the normal pituitary gland, as desired in the management of advanced carcinoma. In attempting to accomplish with radiation the equivalent of a hypophysectomy, Kelly et al.[53] have delivered to the normal pituitary tissue doses of 8100 to 10,000 r on a protracted basis without inducing appreciable physiologic disturbances or significant microscopic evidence of morphologic modifications. Doses of the order of 110,000 to 190,000 reps were required to destroy the anterior lobe of the hypophysis when Rasmussen, Harper and Kennedy[93] bombarded pituitary glands with beta particles by placing Yttrium[90] pellets in the sella turcica of monkeys.

The potential consequences that, in the treatment of intracranial neoplasms, the incidental but inherent irradiation of the normal pituitary gland might have on the mental and physiologic development of children so exposed are a legitimate concern. Any fear in that respect might be dissipated by considering the long-term results that will be presented for 119 children whose pituitary glands inevitably were irradiated 5 to 25 years ago in the treatment of primary brain tumors.

The close proximity of the eyes to the intracranial content is such that they are often irradiated to some degree in the treatment of primary or other intracranial tumors. The eye in its entirety might tolerate fairly well the doses of radiation that it may receive in such circumstances. However, the possibility of late postradiation cataract must not be overlooked and ought to be prevented if possible without omitting to treat adequately a malignant intracranial tumor which otherwise may take the patient's life away if not treated successfully. The dosage levels which may induce postradiation cataracts as published by Merriam[78] should be most useful for guidance.

EFFECTS OF RADIATION THERAPY ON PRIMARY MALIGNANT INTRACRANIAL NEOPLASMS

Assessment of Radiosensitivity of Brain Tumors

The degree of radiosensitivity of primary intracranial tumors is variable from one histologic type to another and, for tumors within the same histopathologic group, from one individual case to another. This general statement indicates that radiosensitivity is a biological character which is difficult to evaluate fully regarding the effects of irradiation in the treatment of intracranial neoplasms. Perhaps that accounts for the controversial if not contradictory opinions which have often been expressed in relation to the role of radiation therapy in the management of some of the primary brain tumors.

If the degrees of radiosensitivity could be predicted or the results of irradiation evaluated solely on the physical intensity of irradiation based upon the time-dose-volume factors, it would simplify greatly the problem of assessing the response of brain tumors to irradiation. However it is not that simple, since the response of apparently identical brain tumors varies considerably in relation to comparable intensity of irradiation.

Besides the physical factors just mentioned, the radiosensitivity of brain tumors may be related also to biological factors difficult to fathom and of which we know very little. Biologic reactions, which are outstanding and common to many primary intracranial neoplasms, are growth restraint and tumor regression by degenerative process commonly induced with radiation doses which often exceed the tolerance of normal brain tissue. The accumulated experience of various observers strongly suggests a difference of radiosensitivity at cellular level, for instance in medulloblastomas. Actually, there is a fairly common pattern of response in most histological varieties of primary intracranial tumors, when treated under identical physical conditions of irradiation and within the generally accepted dose tolerance levels for normal brain tissue adjacent to irradiated tumors.

Radiosensitivity of Different Gliomas and Other Intracranial Tumors

The relative degrees of radiosensitivity of brain tumors have emerged gradually from common patterns of clinical improvement and have been confirmed by tests consisting mostly of neuroradiologic examinations demonstrating objective evidence of tumor regression. Histological verification of postradiation regression is rather scanty and histologic proof of total disappearance of irradiated brain tumors is indeed rare and difficult to obtain.

It is our opinion that adequate radiation therapy may be effective in all types of glioma, but not to the same degree in all. Medulloblastomas always seem to be radiosensitive as they invariably appear to regress. There is universal agreement that medulloblastomas are the most radiosensitive of all primary intracranial tumors, although they may be curable only in a proportion which varies from one to 2 out of 5. Malignant ependymomas or ependyblastomas are also very radiosensitive and usually exhibit a higher degree of radio-curability than medulloblastomas, as at least 1 of 2 patients with ependymal cell tumors may be expected to survive 5 years or longer. Lindgren[68] has reported healing of the primary tumor, verified histologically, in 4 cases of medulloblastoma and in 1 case of ependymoma. He emphasized that, in spite of sizable differences in tumor doses, there was no necrosis observed in the healthy cerebral tissue immediately surrounding the tumor in any of those cases.

Gliomas originating from the astrocytes represent by far the majority of the gliomatous tumors. Considerable differences of opinion are prevailing in respect to the relative degrees of radiosensitivity within the broad group of malignant gliomas generally regarded as being of astrocytic origin. Glioblastoma multiforme is the most malignant of all intracranial neoplasms and it is considered as radioresistant by most people. Although it is recognized that its radiosensitivity is low, in our experience, glioblastoma seems to respond to radiation therapy in the majority of cases even though its growth restraint is usually of short duration. Consequently radiocurability of glioblastomas is poor, but there is always the odd case which will respond better than anticipated, if adequately irradiated, so that patients may survive for 5 years or longer in the proportion of 1 out of 15[14]. For a long time the only proven case on record in which a glioblastoma has been destroyed by irradiation was reported by Pennybacker and Russell[87]. Lindgren[68] has reported 2 cases of glioblastoma in which at autopsy no residual tumor was found at the site of the primary tumor, but there was necrosis in its place and this necrosis was involving the surrounding brain tissue also.

In the intermediate type of astrocytoma, which appears in our own material as unclassified malignant glioma, tumors usually show a moderate degree of radiosensitivity. Results indicate that we may anticipate that approximately 1 of 3 malignant gliomas classified in this group will remain under control for 5 years or longer[14]. Lindgren[68] has reported no residual tumor following irradiation of one astrocytoma of the intermediate type, but necrosis was present at the site of the primary tumor.

The low grade and well-differentiated astrocytomas are generally considered as tumors of low radiosensitivity. Our opinion differs appreciably. In contrasting survival rates between a first group of patients who were believed not to require irradiation following surgical removal and a second group of patients irradiated postoperatively because of evidence of residual tumor, it appears clearly that our results at 5 years and 10 years after treatment have been superior in the group of irradiated patients[15].

The usually slowly growing oligodendroglioma and the low malignancy oligodendroglioblastoma are also tumors of limited radiosensitivity. When irradiated the oligodendroglial tumors require doses which approach or sometimes exceed the dose tolerance of the normal brain tissue. Adequate protracted irradiation seems helpful in controlling tumors of this histologic type when removed incompletely or showing malignant characters. In the oligodendroglioma group of patients adequately irradiated postoperatively, our results have shown that in 1 of 2 patients the condition has remained under control for 5 years or longer.

Outside of the glioma group, practically all other histologic types of intracranial tumors are capable of responding in some degree to radiation therapy. However, the degree of radiosensitivity is variable and it must be determined for each individual group of tumors. Only in a limited way should the selection of cases suitable for irradiation be made purely on the basis of known radiosensitivity. The selection should be made primarily on the basis of other factors that will be presented in the next chapter in which indications and contraindications for radiation therapy will be discussed.

Histopathologic Effects of Radiation Therapy on Primary Brain Tumors

The histologic assessment of the degree of tumor damage as a direct radiobiologic effect on gliomas is difficult. When gliomas which have been treated by irradiation are examined histologically, the amount of tissue changes which may be attributed to radiation therapy alone can hardly be differentiated from variable degrees of necrosis, hemorrhage and vascular changes which often occur spontaneously in the non-irradiated tumors, particularly in the most malignant.

Nessa[80] endeavored to determine the histologic effects of radiation therapy on primary brain tumors by comparing biopsy material obtained before irradiation with postradiation tissue procured at a later operation or else at autopsy. Reduction in the number of mitotic figures and decrease in the cellularity of tumor tissue, increase in the amount of fibrous material with fibrous replacement of the tumor elements, and thickening of the walls of the blood vessels are all histopathologic changes which may be identified in cerebral gliomata. Such changes can be interpreted either as secondary to irradiation or else as evidence of degenerative changes which may occur spontaneously without previous irradiation.

Freed and Davidoff[36] stated that the histopathologic changes seen in some gliomas, following irradiation, can be attributed mainly to the roentgen therapy administered. They believed that the intensity of the changes induced in tumors was not always proportional to the dose of radiation administered. It was their opinion that the histologic changes observed in some gliomas subsequently to irradiation would be called postradiation effects in tumors located in other parts of the body. But, they also recognized that identical changes often occur in gliomas without irradiation. Necrosis, areas of calcification, atypical giant cells, fibroblasts, hyalinization in the walls of blood vessels may all be seen in gliomas not previously irradiated. Yet, the same tissue changes, when found elsewhere but in irradiated tumors of the central nervous system, are usually considered indicative of radiation effects on the tumor itself.

Nearly all the histopathologic studies on the effects of radiation therapy on primary brain tumors reveal consistently the finding of microscopic evidence of residual tumor cells at the site of the primary neoplastic lesion. Whether these cells may be viable or not is a biological character which cannot be determined with any degree of certainty from their morphology. Our experience coincides with that of the majority of observers (Peirce and Bouchard).[85] From a series of 130 patients with glioblastomas, irradiated with tumor doses averaging 6500 r up to 7500 r in approximately 6 to 8 weeks, tumor cells were found at the site of the primary neoplasm in all cases reoperated upon (24 cases) or autopsied (30 cases). Recently, I have reviewed the autopsy findings in 63 of 564 patients who were exposed to intensive irradiation for all types of primary intracranial neoplasms, and there is not a single case in which complete disappearance of all tumor cells has been observed.

Pennybacker and Russell[87] have reported the first case of glioblastoma which at autopsy showed microscopic evidence of complete disappearance of tumor cells, a finding attributed by them to treatment with large doses of radiation.

In an outstanding study on the tolerance of brain tissue and the sensitivity of brain tumors to irradiation, Lindgren[68] has reported 10 cases in which no residual tumor cells could be found at autopsy. His study is based upon 71 cases of intracranial gliomas treated with radiation which were carefully studied at post mortem and of which 18 proved to be highly informative. Autopsy findings revealed no residual tumor cells at the primary site in 5 cases (4 medulloblastomas, 1 ependymoma), in which only 2 had been subjected to craniotomy and 1 of the 2 had had a partial extirpation; the adjacent cerebral tissue appeared to be relatively healthy. In the 5 other cases (2 glioblastomas, 1 intermediate type of glioma, 1 medulloblastoma and 1 pinealoma) irradiated following partial surgical removal in all but one, no tumor cells were found at the primary site, but the space previously occupied by the primary tumor was filled with necrotic material. He pointed out that the power of brain tissue to form connective tissue is low so that disintegrating tumor masses tend to remain in situ as necrotic material. The glial reaction is slow to appear and the result eventually is a glial scar or a cystic defect. However, Lindgren believes that, when major surgery has preceded irradiation, arachnoid tissue inserted in the brain may stimulate connective tissue cicatrisation.

Lindgren,[68] in the same report, has presented 6 cases in which sizable doses of radiation had induced massive brain necrosis but had failed to destroy the primary gliomata as residual tumor cells were found at its site.

In final analysis, there are only a few cases on record in which there is unquestionable histologic proof that cerebral gliomata have disappeared completely following irradiation. Most of the microscopic studies of intracranial tumors which had received radiation doses considered adequate (doses approaching and occasionally exceeding the tolerance of normal brain tissue) have revealed the presence of residual tumor cells at the site of the primary brain tumor.

The radiobiologic effects on primary intracranial gliomata and other neoplasms, following irradiation of adequate intensity, can be best appraised on the basis of the immediate clinical results observed during the course of treatment and subsequent months, and far more from the long-term results estimated by the survival and recovery rates.

CARCINOGENESIS FOLLOWING RADIATION THERAPY OF PRIMARY INTRACRANIAL NEOPLASMS

Malignant Gliomas Induced by Radiation

The induction by ionizing radiation of malignant gliomas is one potential radiobiologic effect which to my knowledge has not been demonstrated as yet. It appears that malignant transformation of glial cells in response to the carcinogenic stimulation of ionizing radiation might be a rare phenomenon if it ever occurs. There are numerous reports on postirradiation damage involving glial cells in experimental animals but I am not aware of any report on gliomas induced by radiation.

Postirradiation Fibrosarcomas of Brain

In recent years, considerable interest was aroused by a few reports of malignant mesenchymal tumors, mostly fibrosarcomas, which developed intracranially at the site or in the vicinity of primary intracranial neoplasms which had been treated by irradiation with or without surgical procedures.

Noetzli and Malamud[81] reported a case of fibrosarcoma which developed within the brain tissue of a patient who had been previously irradiated following the surgical removal of a large cerebellar medulloblastoma. The patient had remained well for nearly 8 years when she developed clinical signs which were attributed to recurrence of her medulloblastoma. She died a few months later and at autopsy there was no evidence of medulloblastoma, but a large fibrosarcoma was found arising from the posterior part of the left cerebral hemisphere.

On the occasion of that report, Noetzli and Malamud[81] reviewed the literature in respect to postirradiation fibrosarcoma of brain. They quoted Chasmar et al.[19] who are of the opinion that fibrosarcoma is the commonest form of cancer to develop in previously irradiated connective tissue. On that basis and in the belief that primary fibrosarcoma of the brain is rare, Noetzli and Malamud[81] have suggested that the malignant mesenchymal tumor found in their case could have been induced by radiation. The finding of certain histological changes, which are commonly attributed to effects of irradiation, was also used in support of their opinion.

It is interesting to note that in a few cases of postirradiation fibrosarcoma which were reported individually by Mann and co-workers[73], by Zulch[128] and also by Russell and Rubinstein[103] the mesenchymal tumors had arisen in the dura at the site of the previous surgical procedure and irradiation. In the 3 cases reported by Terry, Hyams, and Davidoff[113] the sarcomatous tumors also developed at the site of previous operation and irradiation as the sarcomas arose within the primary pituitary chromophobe adenomas for which they had been treated. The salient feature in the case of Noetzli and Malamud[81] is that the fibrosarcoma was apparently unrelated to either the site of surgical tumor removal or at the level of the dura but developed within an area which had been indirectly irradiated in the course of radiation therapy. Noetzli and Malamud[81] stated that the time interval between irradiation and the development of fibrosarcomas intracranially has averaged 6 to 11 years.

Not a single case of intracranial sarcoma, subsequent to irradiation with or without surgical procedure, has been identified and observed in our own clinical material. Our experience, however, comprises the case of a 32-year-old patient who developed an extracranial fibrosarcoma exactly 5 years after surgical removal and postoperative irradiation of an astrocytoma located in the right frontal lobe. The dose of radiation received by tissues in that anatomic location was nearly 4000 rads in 51 days. The sarcomatous lesion arose from beneath the scalp at the site of the right frontal cranioplasty. The initial treatment of this fibrosarcoma consisted of local excision. The tumor recurred 1 year later when it was excised radically, and it has remained under control ever since (3 years). The pathological sections were reviewed by Dr. H. M. Zimmerman[125] who expressed the view that the tumor might represent sarcomatous growth whose development had been stimulated by irradiation. Experimentally, Zimmerman and Arnold[122] using benzpyrene as carcinogenic agents induced 14 gliomas, 9 fibrosarcomas and 2 extracranial fibrosarcomas.

Incidence of Spontaneous and Postirradiation Brain Sarcomas

The incidence of intracranial and extracranial fibrosarcomas induced by irradiation cannot be denied but it must be extremely low. Fibrosarcomas have been demonstrated intracranially following surgical treatment alone. Fibrosarcomas have been reported by Feigin and Gross[33] to arise spontaneously within glioblastomas which at the time of diagnosis had not been subjected to any surgical procedure nor exposed to radiation. Kernohan and Uihlein[56] have reported 96 primary intracranial fibrosarcomas of which 27 have had roentgen therapy following surgical removal of some or part of the tumors. They have encountered no occurrence of malignant mesodermal neoplasms following therapeutic irradiation of their cases of brain tumors. Zulch[128] reported 1 case of fibrosarcoma which developed approximately 8 years after surgical removal and irradiation of an ependymoma. This fibrosarcoma was found growing along the entire suture line in the dura. Apparently this is the only case in which irradiation with conventional doses might have provoked the tumor growth of an intracranial fibrosarcoma in the series of Zulch[128] which comprises 6000 intracranial tumors of which there were 1079 meningiomas and 30 fibrosarcomas.

From the evidence reported above, it appears that carcinogenesis following radiation therapy of primary intracranial neoplasms is very low, indeed rare. The carcinogenic effect of ionizing radiation may have resulted in humans in an extremely small number of malignant intracranial or extracranial mesenchymal neoplasms which may be considered as the result of radiobiologic effect. As yet, evidence of intracranial gliomas presumably related to exposure to ionizing radiation is not available.

3

Role of Ionizing Radiation in the Treatment of Primary Intracranial Neoplasms

THE ROLE of ionizing radiation as a therapeutic agent in the control of primary malignant intracranial tumors is determined by its power to restrain and induce regression of growth, and by its contribution to the preservation of life and recovery of function. Unquestionable clinical and histologic evidence has demonstrated that the majority of primary intracranial tumors are radiosensitive to some degree. Medulloblastomas are the most sensitive to radiation in contrast with glioblastomas whose radiosensitivity is minimal and radiocurability very low.

As yet, surgery and radiation, used alone or jointly, are the only methods of treatment which have accomplished lasting results or apparent cures in the control of intracranial neoplasms.

When radiation therapy is used for primary intracranial neoplasms, it is mostly in combination with surgical treatment, as a postoperative procedure. Surgical methods are and continue to be the most important in the management of those tumors. Various surgical techniques are used to obtain tissue for histopathologic studies and arrive at a firm diagnosis. The relief of increased intracranial pressure by shunt or other surgical decompression means is imperative in many cases, especially prior to initiation of radiation therapy and particularly when it is intended to use irradiation alone for treatment. In the majority of the gliomas compressing adjacent structures, craniotomy and partial removal of neoplastic tissue by suction or electrocoagulation is indicated primarily. However, surgical removal no longer needs to be radical since neurosurgeons know that they can preserve or restore function by partial removal only and may depend upon postoperative radiation therapy to complete treatment.

Certain types of tumors can be removed surgically in toto. Complete removal can be accomplished in cerebellar astrocytomas, meningiomas and hemangioblastomas. In such cases the rate of recurrence is low and postoperative irradiation is not indicated.

Chemotherapy used systemically has failed so far to prove its value, as

56

no particular drug has demonstrated as yet definite specificity or affinity for tumors arising from the central nervous system. Alkylating drugs, antibiotics, antimetabolites and other chemotherapeutic agents have been reported to induce moderate but transitory improvement when administered by arterial perfusion or infusion techniques.

INDICATIONS FOR RADIATION THERAPY

The indications for radiation therapy in the management of primary intracranial tumors must be clearly enunciated. All cases of primary intracranial neoplasms are not requiring radiation therapy. Irradiation should be considered when a case presents certain requirements. In our opinion, the indications for irradiation bring the patients into 5 categories:

1) Patients, whose tumor has been treated surgically but could not be extirpated completely, should receive adequate postoperative irradiation.

Although certain tumors may be removed satisfactorily, time and experience have shown that, in most gliomata, actual removal in toto rarely occurs. For this reason additional treatment with irradiation is required following operation in the majority of gliomas.

2) Patients, whose brain tumor was not removed at the time of craniotomy and surgical exploration, must be treated by irradiation alone.

In this second category of patients, a biopsy is obtained in some so that a definite histologic diagnosis might be established, although this is not always the case. This occurs when a tumor is located in a highly critical area like the mid-brain, the pons, the motor area of the cerebral cortex, because its surgical extirpation is then considered too hazardous for the patient's life or for a useful recovery.

3) Patients, who are not considered suitable cases for craniotomy and surgical removal, should be treated with radiation only, once a histologic proof of brain tumor has been established from tissue biopsy.

Cases in that category may be medulloblastomas, cerebellar sarcomas, pinealomas or other mid-brain tumors, and occasionally gliomas involving the cerebral motor area.

4) Those presenting with definite clinical evidence of a tumor growing in the pons or brain stem should be treated with radiation only, even without histologic proof.

Too many patients are denied treatment for tumors located in such critical regions of the central nervous system. No attempt at surgical removal is made because of the high operative mortality rate. Irradiation is excluded because histological proof is lacking. And yet, the diagnosis is established on otherwise sound evidence.

Patients in this category should not go untreated and be abandoned to a rapid lethal fate since postmortem examinations consistently have demonstrated the presence of primary tumors, mostly gliomata. I do not think that one must insist on a definite histopathologic diagnosis of brain stem tumor and I believe one is fully justified to initiate radiation therapy without it.

Treatment by irradiation alone is applicable to a minority of patients with primary intracranial tumors (indications 2, 3, and 4). Actually there are only 16.8 per cent of our patients for whom radiation therapy only was indicated and utilized.

5) Those whose tumor has recurred after a surgical removal, considered complete at the time of operation, should have external radiation therapy unless another operation is considered more advisable.

Irradiation may be preferable in recurrent brain tumors, providing increased pressure can be controlled adequately. Further surgery is rather indicated for cystic tumors and some meningiomas.

CONTRAINDICATIONS TO RADIATION THERAPY

Contraindications to the treatment of intracranial tumors by irradiation may be absolute and decisive when they preclude the use of radiation therapy in a majority of cases. They may be relative and transitory when they merely prevent initiation of irradiation until certain prohibitive conditions have been corrected satisfactorily or removed completely.

Absolute Contraindications

1) Inadequate diagnosis or localization of a primary intracranial tumor.

2) Diffuse degenerative encephalitis such as reported and identified in toxic conditions like uremia or severe anoxia, or observed occasionally in lymphosarcoma.

Diffuse gliosis involving one or both cerebral hemispheres may at times simulate an astrocytoma, and it should not be treated with radiation therapy. Cerebral atrophy, either unilateral or bilateral, may contraindicate the use of radiation therapy or at least should caution against the administration of dosage which may exceed the minimum level of brain tolerance.

3) Recurrence of a brain tumor, without adequate proof of neoplastic reactivation, on a presumptive basis, irrelevant of the treatment procedures previously used.

4) Previous intensive irradiation of an intracranial tumor should preclude the use of further irradiation in the event of neoplastic reactivation, because of the considerable risk of postradiation damage and brain necrosis when a second course is administered.

Exceptionally, we have re-irradiated a brain tumor, providing that satisfactory evidence of tumor reactivation was available, that the patient had made a good recovery and that the period of remission from initial irradiation to the time of recurrence was not less than 6 months and preferably longer. It must be emphasized that recurrence of a brain tumor may easily be simulated by distention of residual cystic areas or a hemorrhage within the previously treated region.

Adequate re-irradiation of an intracranial neoplasm is always hazardous in regard to postradiation injury, a risk which must be clearly understood and accepted by all concerned. Some patients have tolerated a second tumor dose as large as the initial one without subsequent complications, but this is unpredictable. I wish to recall at this point that our only case of postradiation brain necrosis has developed 3 years after re-irradiation of a sarcoma which had recurred nearly 3 years after initial treatment. When a second course of radiation therapy is administered adequate protraction of dose is imperative.

5) Routine or prophylactic postoperative radiation therapy is not advocated for tumors which ordinarily can be eradicated completely by surgery, when the neurosurgeon feels certain that he has extirpated the neoplasm in toto.

This contraindication must be determined for each individual patient. It mostly applies to the "benign" types qualified by Horrax as favorable tumors, which consist of the majority of meningeal tumors in adults, and of the cerebellar cystic astrocytomas and the few hemangiomatous cysts in children.

Relative Contraindications

1) Uncontrolled severe intracranial pressure with probable cerebral edema, until the increased pressure is under control through adequate and persistent decompressive measures including, if necessary, suitable medication such as diuretics and steroids, should be considered a relative contraindication.

Patients should not be denied radiation therapy if their condition appears critical providing that their intracranial pressure can be controlled. In many instances, patients who were accepted for treatment despite their critical condition eventually recovered and enjoyed long useful survival.

2) Lack of histopathologic diagnosis to indicate the exact type of an intracranial tumor, when this can be determined without undue risk for the patient's life, should be considered a relative contraindication.

It is always desirable to know the exact histopathologic diagnosis because it permits to anticipate what the effect of treatment might be, depending upon the type of tumor to be irradiated, its location, its extent, its recognized degree of radiosensitivity and the accumulated experience with results of radiation therapy.

TREATMENT PLANNING

Once the above indications and contraindications for the use of radiation therapy have been discussed in consultation with the neurosurgeon and the neurologist, and it has been agreed that irradiation is advisable for a patient with intracranial neoplasm, an adequate plan of treatment must be prepared.

Tumor Localization and Technical Approach

Accurate localization and demarcation of the tumor-bearing area is essential. This is usually accomplished by making a topographic reconstitution of each tumor. For this most important part of treatment planning, one must use fully all the information available from the clinical picture, the neuroradiologic and many other special investigative examinations which may be indicated, together with the operative findings of the neurosurgeon. All that information is required to assist in determining the proper size and location of the fields and ascertain that each external beam of radiation be directed through the entire tumor.

Pin-point localization of primary brain tumors should be avoided because of the risk of not irradiating part of the tumor and jeopardizing a patient's chances for a cure. The opposite approach, consisting of intensive irradiation of the entire intracranial content without specific reasons, is an extreme solution to the problem of accurate localization and beam direction.

Once we are satisfied that the location and extent of a brain tumor is confined to part of one cerebral hemisphere, a suitable technical plan of irradiation is devised for each patient individually. It is essential to circumscribe the tumor from every direction. This can be accomplished most efficiently by an arrangement of fields such that growth may be controlled primarily in both antero-posterior and vertical direction: opposing beams of megavoltage radiation are directed from the front and from the back of the calvarium through the affected hemisphere only. Tumor extension in the transverse direction towards and possibly beyond mid-line is the rationale for lateral fields being placed not only on the homolateral side of the tumor-bearing area but on the contralateral side as well (Plate 1, a and b.). Field sizes vary from 6 x 8 to 6 x 10 cm. in the antero-posterior direction, and 8 x 8 to 10 x 12 cm.laterally. The wedge filter pair arrangement proposed by Patterson[83] for small field irradiation of eccentrically placed tumors would seem to be most suitable in the treatment of small and well-circumscribed tumors, particularly when located in the tips of the frontal or parietal lobes. Occasionally tumors identical in size and location might be small enough to be adequately irradiated with a single electron beam of very high energy, in the 30 to 50 Mev. range.

PLATE 1

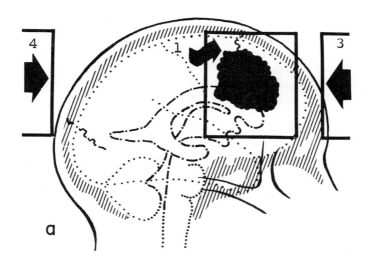

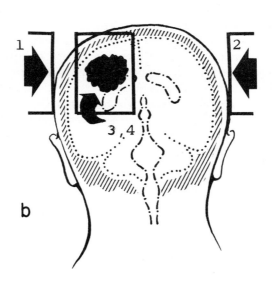

Glioma Confined to One Cerebral Hemisphere. Position of Fields and Beam Direction

The natural tendency of certain cerebral gliomata to spread by direct invasion along known anatomic paths and even cross mid-line at times has already been mentioned, because this must be taken into consideration in the planning of treatment by irradiation. It has been demonstrated by Concannon, Kramer and Berry[21] that brain tumors are almost invariably larger and more extensive than suspected by clinical and roentgenologic examination. Concannon *et al.* have concluded that there is no place for small or medium volume radiation therapy in the more malignant gliomata. It means that localized irradiation can be effective only insofar as the radiotherapist in planning treatment is reasonably certain that the fields will be large enough to include all of the intracranial neoplasm in each individual case.

When there is evidence that a hemispheral glioma extends beyond mid-line or there is a suspicion that the tumor might actually cross over, the field size and arrangement in the antero-posterior direction must be such that the beam of radiation will include part or all of the opposite hemisphere (Plate 2, a and b), including the third ventricle. In some cases, the tumor is so extensive that the entire intracranial content may have to be irradiated homogeneously.

In medulloblastomas, the entire intracranial content must always be irradiated because of their natural tendency to spread to the ventricles and all the subarachnoid spaces within the skull and the spinal canal. This illustrates the importance of knowing the histopathology of a tumor for adequate planning of its treatment with ionizing radiation. The treatment technique in medulloblastomas will be discussed and illustrated (Plate 3) further in this book, in the section devoted to the medulloblastomas.

Treatment planning of tumors growing in the mid-brain and pontine regions usually depends more upon the critical anatomic location of the primary tumor than its exact pathology. These are located in highly critical parts of the central nervous system which commonly are not safely accessible for biopsy or surgical extirpation. The technique of irradiation will be presented in the chapter on Results of Treatment of Gliomatous Tumors involving the Mid-brain and the Brain Stem (Plates 4, 5 and 6).

Sources of Ionizing Radiation or Particles Available

In treatment planning, one must select the most suitable source of ionizing radiation. Important technical and clinical factors must be considered. It is essential to possess an adequate knowledge and interpretation of the potential radiobiological effects on the normal central nervous system as well as on each type of intracranial neoplasm.

The selection of the most suitable and appropriate sources of ionizing radiation for the treatment of intracranial neoplasm presents virtually no problem. In our opinion the advantages of external irradiation are definitely superseding those of internal irradiation.

PLATE 2

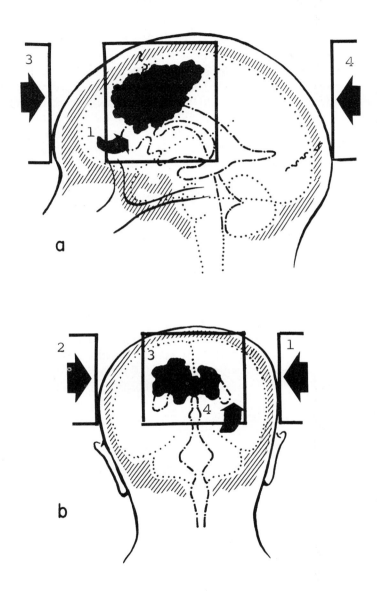

Glioma of Left Frontal Lobe Crossing Mid-line to Right Hemisphere. Position of Fields and Beam Direction

Radioactive Isotopes Used Internally. Internal irradiation of intracranial malignancies with radioisotopes administered either orally or parenterally has been attempted by many. For treatment purposes, no isotope so far has shown a significant tendency to accumulate in intracranial neoplasms in sufficient concentration to induce any appreciable therapeutic effect.

Certain natural isotopes, however, have been found to have a special affinity for rapidly growing brain tumors. These natural isotopes, in particular Boron[10] and Lithium[6], absorb slow neutrons readily and then disintegrate to give short-range radiation in situ. Godwin, Farr, Sweet and Robertson[42] have treated 10 patients with this method, using the intense neutron beam from the Brookhaven pile, while Boron[10] was administered as borax by intravenous injection. The results were inconclusive. From a practical standpoint this is a therapeutic approach which could only be used in the few centers where an atomic pile is available.

Direct intracranial insertion of radioactive isotopes into the tumor-bearing area has been utilized by a few investigators in the treatment of inoperable brain tumors in humans. Beta radiation emitters, especially radioactive gold seeds, were implanted directly into the tumors. Talairach, Ruggiero, Aboulker and David[111] have reported their experience with radiogold seeds in the treatment of 5 inoperable brain tumors. Kerr, Schwartz and Seaman[58] have used intrathecal injections of Au^{198} in a clinical trial on 11 selected patients with hopeless malignant tumors of the brain. They showed that the distribution of radiation effect involved mainly the most superficial portions of the cerebrum, the cerebellum and the most caudal portion of the cord so that additional roentgen therapy needed to be administered to the primary tumor. Kerr *et al.* concluded that the primary tumor could be treated best with x-rays and that Au^{198} could serve to irradiate circulating tumor cells in the cerebrospinal fluid and small implants in the subarachnoid spaces.

Ionizing Radiation Beams. Direct intracranial exposure of a tumor to a beam of low energy X-radiation has been accomplished by introducing the x-ray tube through an open craniotomy. This proved to be a rather complicated technical procedure to perform during a surgical operation. From the radiobiological standpoint, the administration to the brain of a large dose of radiation in a single acute exposure seems to be rather undesirable in humans.

Beams of ionizing radiation which can be applied externally and properly aimed at intracranial neoplasms are currently available from a variety of sources such that the optimum quality of radiation can be selected readily. In the last 10 to 15 years the opportunity to pass from kilovoltage to megavoltage, over a wide range of energy levels, has contributed to stimulate further interest and investigation in the treatment of malignant intracranial tumors.

The quality of radiation required may be provided by the transformation of electrical energy into ionizing radiation of the pre-selected energy level, from 10 Kv to 70 Mev or higher. Thus X-radiation is currently generated in x-ray tubes, linear accelerators and betatrons.

Radioactive elements artificially produced in atomic piles are now used in the making of teletherapy units and have become the most important sources of ionizing radiation beams. The designing and production of teletherapy units containing several kilocuries of Cobalt[60] have made high energy radiation accessible to all in compact and readily serviceable units. The creation in Canada of Cobalt[60] radiation therapy units has proved to be a technical advancement of considerable practical significance. Cesium[137] therapy units have also been designed and made available, but their range of usefulness has remained somewhat limited.

The only natural radioactive element used in teletherapy units has been radium whose supply was limited and cost prohibitive. Radium "bombs" have always been low intensity units, which had to be used at short distance and limited to small volume irradiation. The largest radium bomb ever made was loaded with 50 milligrams of radium, a fabulous quantity of radioactive material at the time but a very small amount by today's standards as kilocuries are loaded in Cobalt[60] units.

Beams of High Energy Particles. Sources of high energy radiation such as the linear accelerator and the betatron may also be designed to produce beams of electrons. These negatively charged ionizing particles have some physical properties whose potential radiobiological effects are under investigation.

Other high energy particles are also used in therapeutic trials on advanced tumors of the central nervous system. Those high energy particles consist of protons, neutrons, deuterons, alpha particles and mesons.

Selection of Most Suitable Sources of Radiation for the Treatment of Brain Tumors

Evidence available at present time suggests that ionizing radiation beams used externally may provide most desirable radiobiological effects and clinical results when used judiciously in the management of brain tumors. Slight differences of opinion still persist as to which may be the optimum quality of radiation to be selected for that purpose.

Our experience has demonstrated conclusively that primary intracranial neoplasms can be treated adequately and safely with ionizing radiation generated at energy level of 200 to 250 Kv. Kilovoltage radiation is currently designating this quality of radiation which is corresponding to so-called conventional or orthovoltage deep x-ray therapy.

Megavoltage high energy radiation offers certain technical, biological and clinical advantages which must be considered and utilized for the benefit of patients. Survival and recovery rates, however, may not necessarily be superior to those attained with kilovoltage radiation.

The main technical advantage of megavoltage radiation in the treatment of intracranial neoplasms consists of a greater penetrating power such that better depth dose distribution can be obtained. This advantage applies particularly when crossfiring in the antero-posterior direction through deep intracranial neoplasms or when tumors of small volume are irradiated. The increased depth dose is combined with lesser absorption by bone, so that the use of high energy radiation should minimize the potential danger of postradiation aseptic bone necrosis which could develop in the calvarium or in the base of the skull. The radiobiological effects on the other intervening cephalic structures should be attenuated with high energy radiation. Scalp reactions should rarely exceed the degree of mild erythema so that late changes consisting of telangiectasis and atrophy will not be observed. The incidence of permanent epilation of the scalp has diminished markedly, an advantage which is not of major importance but not negligible.

Because of the multiple advantages just mentioned above, megavoltage radiation should be used in the treatment of intracranial tumors in preference to kilovoltage radiation. We have increasingly utilized the high energy radiation of Cobalt[60] teletherapy sources since 1955, to the extent that we are now using it exclusively for the irradiation of intracranial neoplasms. All tumor doses recommended hereafter for the treatment of different types of intracranial tumors are expressed in rads and represent the minimal dose of radiation energy absorbed in the tumor itself from Cobalt[60] radiation beams.

After 10 years of experience with the use of Cobalt[60] radiation beams in the treatment of intracranial neoplasms, I must state that we have not observed as yet any significant difference in survival and recovery rates, that could be attributed to the use of megavoltage in preference to kilovoltage radiation therapy. Our experience in the treatment of primary intracranial tumors with kilovoltage X-radiation is such that we should be capable of making adequate comparison and assessment of relative differences in therapeutic effects, if any, between the two respective qualities of radiation.

Betatrons generating ionizing radiation beams at 20 to 30 Mev or more are providing radiation of higher energy still. It seems that most of those who have used radiation in that range of quality for the treatment of cerebral gliomata have developed the impression that the results observed are superior to those produced with conventional 200 to 250 Kv radiation. Arnold, Bailey, Harvey and Haas[3] have so stated in relation to their results in the treatment of glioblastoma multiforme with 23 Mev x-rays. In the opinion of Jones[49] the main advantage of supervoltage irradiation is seen in the treatment of localized tumors of the third ventricle.

Mitchell[79] believes that there is no evidence or reason to expect any fundamental difference between the therapeutic effects of 30 Mev and 220 Kv x-rays. But he is of the opinion that the possibility of irradiating adequately certain inoperable malignant intracranial gliomata has been augmented by the use of 30 Mev X-radiation in preference to 220 Kv and 4 Mev x-rays. According to Mitchell, this is due to the improvement in the physical properties of such high energy radiation. One of the physical advantages is the homogeneous penetration of radiation of this quality through dense bone at the base of the skull, resulting in a more even distribution of radiation through the volume of tissue occupied by the glioma. When using 30 Mev radiation, all treatments may be administered through a single field, thus allowing for more accurate irradiation of a small volume of tissue. This physical advantage of a greater accuracy of beam direction in the irradiation of a small volume at 30 Mev may be nullified by the natural characteristic that certain cerebral gliomata possess to extend and infiltrate beyond their apparent limits.

The clinical application of high energy particles consists in a few centers of the treatment of brain tumors with electron beams. It is too early yet to assess the therapeutic effects by comparison with other sources of ionizing particles or with the results of ionizing radiation.

CLINICAL CONSIDERATIONS RELATED TO THE IRRADIATION OF PATIENTS WITH BRAIN TUMORS

Opportune Time for Initiation of Radiation Therapy. This must be determined for each patient in consultation with the neurosurgeon, once it has been agreed that radiation therapy is indicated. Irradiation can begin as soon as it may be administered safely without inducing any significant complication. In postoperative irradiation, treatment is usually initiated approximately 2 weeks after operation, when the scalp incision is well healed and local subcutaneous fluid collection or edema have regressed.

Irradiation of a primary intracranial tumor must not be initiated unless increased intracranial pressure is under control, whether the patient is to be irradiated postoperatively or treated with radiation alone. Decompressive procedures must be established and maintained with effectiveness in all cases in which there is marked increase of intracranial pressure at the onset of treatment.

Once irradiation is initiated, it is important to persist and persevere until treatment has been completed. Occasionally a course of treatment may have to be slowed down and perhaps interrupted for a few days. Irradiation should be resumed as soon as possible and continued as a single course inasmuch as radiation effect is cumulative. In many instances patients have been accepted for irradiation despite their critical condition, and yet many of them have recovered eventually and survived for a long time.

Cerebral Edema. The fear that cerebral edema might develop and become so severe as to cause death must not be so great that a patient will be deprived from adequate radiation therapy when indicated in the management of a primary intracranial tumor. It must be realized that some degree of cerebral edema may be present before treatment is initiated, either because of increased intracranial pressure or due to the size of the tumor itself. Cerebral edema can be aggravated by excessive initial doses of radiation, unless it is first relieved by decompressive surgical procedures or by adequate medication. The risk of lethal cerebral edema may be greater for patients who will be treated with radiation alone, without decompression, than for those exposed to postoperative irradiation after a craniotomy has been performed and the bulk of the tumor removed. Edema may occasionally develop during the initial part of the course of radiation therapy, even after decompression has been accomplished with shunts or other procedures.

Cerebral edema can be identified by aggravation of the neurologic symptoms and signs, particularly by headache of increasing severity. When severe edema develops after completion of treatment, a rare occurrence in our experience, it may simulate reactivation of the tumor growth. From a practical standpoint, in order to obviate any complication from existing or potential cerebral edema, regardless of whether or not the patient has had a decompression prior to treatment, we usually administer only 50 to 100 rads tumor dose through but one port for the first 3 or 4 treatments at the onset of a course of radiation therapy. By protracting total tumor doses of 5000 to 6000 rads or more over a period of 50 to 60 days, complicating cerebral edema has been avoided in nearly all cases.

Radiation Sickness. Such manifestation of systemic reactions to radiation therapy is uncommon in the treatment of intracranial neoplasms when protracted fractionated doses adding up to not more than 800 to 900 rads tumor dose per week are administered. So much so that when a patient vomits under treatment, it is more often related to developing increased intracranial pressure or to some complication other than radiation sickness. When the patient's symptoms cannot be attributed to any other cause but radiation sickness, daily radiation doses should be reduced and ordinary treatment against radiation sickness should be instituted. Symptomatic medication must be used as required.

Importance of Clinical Team. Close collaboration between the neurosurgeon and the therapeutic radiologist is essential during all phases of treatment. It is essential that both the neurosurgeon and the radiation therapist observe the patient closely during the first few days of treatment and, if indicated, they re-assess the case and modify the plan of treatment. The necessity for periodic decompression has become negligible in recent years, probably because of careful planning and cautious administration of radiation therapy. During and after the period of treatment, the physical, psychological and social rehabilitation of each patient must be a constant concern, in order that the quality of their survival be as good as possible and that a high recovery rate be obtained.

4 Overall Results of Treatment of Primary Intracranial Neoplasms Following Surgical Removal Plus Irradiation or Irradiation Alone

THE VALUE of ionizing radiation therapy in the management of primary intracranial neoplasms must be determined from the immediate and late results observed over the years. For that purpose, it is my intention to use our own results to a large extent.

Over a period of 25 years, from 1939 to 1963 inclusive, we have treated with external irradiation 788 patients affected with primary intracranial tumors, of which 668 were classified with the gliomata and 120 or 15.2 per cent with the non-gliomatous tumors (Table 1).

TABLE 1. Primary Intracranial Neoplasms (Adequately Irradiated) Author's Experience over 25 Years, 1939–1963

Type or Location	Number of Cases		
	1939–58	1959–63	Total
Gliomata:			
Glioblastoma	176	49	225
Glioma—unclassified	40	42	82
Astrocytoma	123	54	177
Oligodendroglioma-blastoma	14	3	17
Ependymoma-blastoma	20	3	23
Medulloblastoma	50	13	63
Mid-brain tumors	37	4	41
Brain stem of pontine tumors	34	6	40
	494	174	668
Non-gliomatous Tumors:			
Sarcomas	16	4	20
Meningeal tumors	25	13	38
Vascular tumors	15	7	22
Congenital tumors	8	7	15
Miscellaneous	6	19	25
	70	50	120
TOTAL:	564	224	788

From 1939 to 1958, a period of 20 years, 564 primary brain tumors have been irradiated in our Department under constant conditions. Radiation in the kilovoltage range has been utilized in the treatment of all but 17 tumors, the latter having been exposed to the higher energy of Cobalt[60] radiation. These 564 cases are available for full assessment 5 to 25 years following irradiation. Complete follow-up data have been recorded on each and all of them until the present time, with the exception of one patient with whom communication has ceased after 17 years of close follow-up contact. This patient is a woman who was alive and well when last contacted, 17 years following postoperative irradiation for an ependymoma incompletely removed.

In our series of 564 primary tumors irradiated more than 5 years ago, there are 494 gliomata. Histological confirmation is available in 449 cases, nearly 91 per cent. In the non-gliomatous tumors, histologic proof of diagnosis was obtained in 62 of 70 cases or 88.6 per cent.

The program of radiation therapy applied in the management of the 564 primary intracranial neoplasms under review has consisted of a single series of protracted exposures to kilovoltage radiation (220 to 250 Kv). In general, tumor doses in the range of 5000 to 6000 rads have been delivered over a period of approximately 50 days. During the initial years of our program, various dose levels have been tried. However, it can be stated that the dosage intensity has been fairly consistent through the years, as it has not varied much from an average of 800 to 1000 rads per week (tumor dose) over a period of 6 to 8 consecutive weeks. At the onset of treatment, small daily tumor doses of 50 to 100 rads are used over 4 or 5 days. Subsequently, tumor doses are gradually increased to 150 to 200 rads per sitting, on a basis of 5 treatment-visits per week.

Patients who were not adequately irradiated have been omitted from this series of primary intracranial neoplasms. These were patients who, for some reason or another, had received less than 50 per cent of the average tumor dose usually administered in this series. A total of 45 patients, 19 of whom were more or less terminal with glioblastoma, have been classified as inadequately irradiated on the basis that radiation therapy had little or no opportunity to influence the course of their disease. For all practical purposes, irrespective of the outcome of their illness, such patients had to be regarded as untreated with radiation.

The majority of our patients, (83.2 per cent) were irradiated postoperatively, because of tumors which admittedly had not been removed completely. Exceptionally, postoperative irradiation was administered despite the presumably complete extirpation of a glioma. This was done when relatives insisted for radiation therapy as an extra precautionary procedure against potential tumor recurrence. It seems to be a reasonable thing to do when considering that so many neurosurgeons have expressed the opinion that complete removal of gliomatous tumors is not accomplished too often.

Some patients were not irradiated early after a surgical removal which was believed to be complete, but had radiation therapy later when unquestionable evidence of tumor recurrence was demonstrated. There are 29 patients, or 5.1 per cent of our 564 cases, who were subjected to postoperative irradiation only at the time of recurrence (21 gliomas and 8 malignant meningeal tumors). It must be noted that the period of survival in these cases has been calculated from the onset of irradiation and not from the time of previous surgical management.

IMMEDIATE CLINICAL RESULTS OF RADIATION THERAPY

The significance of the words "immediate results", when these are used in relation with the clinical effects of radiation therapy, must be defined and clearly understood. Immediate results include all clinical changes which may be attributed to ionizing radiation from the onset to completion of exposure, and subsequently over a certain period of time. Immediate effects of irradiation of brain tumors may extend over a period of 6 months or more. The assessment of clinical results on that basis is applicable to cases treated accordingly to the plan of irradiation that we are using in respect to time-dose relations. In the treatment of brain tumors, the immediate clinical effects with either kilovoltage or megavoltage (Cobalt ^{60}) radiation do not appear to differ significantly. Clinical evaluation of immediate results of irradiation must take into account the usual slow rate of recovery and repair of the nervous tissue involved. The total period of "immediate effects" of radiation therapy may be divided into 3 phases, unequal in duration.

The first phase is a latent period which corresponds to the initial 15 to 20 days of treatment. Generally, during this phase, little or no radiobiologic effect may be clinically appreciable. Exceptions are observed, when the latent period is of shorter duration. This commonly happens in the irradiation of highly radiosensitive tumors such as medulloblastomas or poorly differentiated sarcomas in which early and dramatic clinical improvement often occurs. Short latent periods may be observed also in other types of tumors, not so much as result of immediate tumor regression but probably more on account of preexisting edema subsidence following the initial administration of radiation in small doses. It must be realized that cerebral edema may be relieved more often than induced by radiation when it is properly administered.

The second phase is the period of maximum immediate reaction to radiation. The dose accumulation is continued over an additional 35 to 40 days and brings the intracranial tissue reactions to a peak. The height of the reaction may remain at a plateau for 15 to 20 days after completion of irradiation. The transition from the second to the third phase is imperceptible.

The third phase is the period of subsidence of the immediate maximum tissue reactions and major degree of tumor regression. The duration of this phase is indefinite since there seems to be no abrupt termination. The length of the third phase is estimated to be proportional in time to the total period of irradiation and the dose absorbed by the central nervous tissues. The third phase should spread over a period of 60 to 75 days at least. Complete repair or partial regeneration of brain tissue and fiber tracts, disturbed by tumor growth and intensive irradiation, may continue slowly. Clinical evidence of healing with improvement of symptoms and neurologic signs may be detectable as long as 6 to 12 months from the onset of radiation therapy.

The majority of the patients that we have treated postoperatively for primary intracranial tumors, approximately 60 to 65 per cent, were in fairly good clinical condition at the onset of radiation therapy. Among those patients, any improvement that had occurred between surgery and the time that the patient was ready for irradiation must be assessed. Obviously, any amelioration already appreciable at the onset of postoperative irradiation must be attributed almost exclusively to the effects of surgical decompression with or without some degree of tumor removal. When further improvement develops during the initial 2 or 3 weeks of postoperative irradiation, this should not be attributed to radiation therapy but to the previous surgical management, considering that such improvement has occurred during the latent period of radiation effects.

Beyond the first or latent phase of postoperative irradiation of brain tumors the immediate therapeutic effects of radiation should begin to blend with the effects of surgical treatment. In dealing with those patients who had recovered reasonably well at the onset of irradiation, it may be virtually impossible to determine objectively to what extent additional clinical improvement may be related to the radiation therapy administered. Many patients have presented identical favorable clinical courses in the months following surgical management alone, without postoperative irradiation. Considering that patients operated upon for primary intracranial tumors are ordinarily irradiated postoperatively because of residual tumor, any true radiation effect in such cases cannot be determined immediately but only after one year or longer. Such assessment will then be based upon the late results of growth restraint, as demonstrated by absence of recurrence and prolongation of life in comparison with similar cases which were not irradiated postoperatively.

Approximately 35 to 40 per cent of our patients subjected to treatment by irradiation, whether used alone or postoperatively, were in a poor state of health or in critical condition at the onset of irradiation. Any progress made during and following treatment, in terms of improvement of symptoms and good recovery, can be considered as immediate effects attributable to radiation. Gradual improvement has been observed ordinarily during the initial 2, 3 or 4 weeks following the onset of irradiation. In some cases, like in medulloblastomas, cerebellar sarcomas, mid-brain and brain stem tumors a dramatic improvement has often been noted within a few days from the beginning of radiation therapy. In most cases, neurological signs have subsided as patients have regained full consciousness and returned to a fair degree of recovery well before completion of their course of treatment with radiation.

In a few cases little perceptible improvement was observed during the entire course of irradiation administered over periods of 6 to 8 weeks. Subsequent improvement was evidenced some weeks later when the full effect of treatment had been accomplished. Rarely have patients not improved at all during the course of therapy. Regression of the patient's symptoms may continue slowly over a period of 6 to 12 months following irradiation. The degree of improvement can be attributed solely to the effect of radiation. Beyond such a period of time, the value of radiation therapy alone should be demonstrable by a review of the long-term results based upon survival and recovery rates. The same method of evaluation should also reflect the potential efficacy of radiation therapy when administered postoperatively to patients in poor initial condition for tumors of the same histological types.

LENGTH AND QUALITY OF SURVIVAL

Results of treatment of intracranial neoplasms must be assessed under two essential aspects: (1) the length of survival, and (2) the quality of survival expressed by recovery rates. In evaluating the methods of treatment of intracranial tumors, high survival rates are meaningful insomuch as the majority of survivors are capable of resuming an active useful life or at least of caring for themselves, whereas only a low minority are remaining totally disabled, mentally or physically, or both.

The length of survival has been calculated in all our cases from the first day of treatment with radiation. No allowance has been made for correction on account of death resulting from unrelated diseases or accidents. Not a single case had to be recorded as deceased during the first 5, 10 or 15 years following treatment because of lack of follow-up information. I repeat here that our follow-up records are complete to this date for all but one patient who has become untraceable only after 17 years of close follow-up from the time of her treatment.

In evaluating the quality of survival, the degree of clinical recovery is estimated and recorded as good, fair or poor corresponding to a grading in categories I, II or III as shown in Table 2. The quality of survival is good when the patient has returned to an active useful life; it is fair, if some degree of partial disability has persisted more than 3 to 6 months after completion of treatment; it is poor, when total disability has developed and the patient has remained completely incapable physically or mentally, or both. A valid and objective assessment of the degree of recovery has been relatively facile in the present series because of the accumulated clinical follow-up information which could lend itself to very little subjective interpretation.

Degree of Recovery in Patients Who Survived Under 5 Years

It is important to know the degree of recovery obtained during the major part of the survival of the 368 patients who lived less than 5 years following irradiation. These represent 65 per cent of the 564 patients that we have irradiated for primary intracranial neoplasms.

Only 9 per cent of the 368 patients who have survived less than 5 years after irradiation have shown no improvement whatsoever, regardless of the length of survival of individual patients, whether it was just a few months or a few years. It is estimated that 19 per cent have remained with some degree of partial disability. It is significant that 72 per cent were well for the major part of their survival. This overall assessment of the quality of survival among those who have survived less than 5 years has applied to all age groups of patients, both adults and children. Such results are gratifying enough to encourage and stimulate anyone to continue to use radiation therapy when indicated in the management of primary intracranial neoplasms.

Long-Term Survival and Recovery Rates

Results Following Adequate Irradiation Used Postoperatively or Alone. Our overall results, based upon 564 primary intracranial neoplasms of all types, have been tabulated in such a way that both survival and recovery rates are presented side by side in Table 2. All patients had the opportunity to survive and be observed clinically not less than 5 years subsequent to adequate irradiation, administered postoperatively or alone. Obviously, the number of those whose treatment dates back far enough to allow survivals to be assessed 10, 15 or 20 years, up to 25, after treatment, is decreasing with each 5-year period (Table 2). For instance, of the 564 patients treated more than 5 years ago, 111 were treated between 1939 and 1943, and it is interesting to note that 21 or 19 per cent of those 111 potential 20-year survivors have actually survived over 20 years.

Many are skeptical regarding the quality of survival of patients who have been irradiated for primary brain tumors and have survived over long periods of time. In order to arrive at true recovery rates, expessed by the percentage of those whose recovery grading was good, fair or poor, more than 5, 10, 15 or 20 years after irradiation of their brain and intracranial

TABLE 2. Primary Intracranial Neoplasms
Long-Term Survival and Recovery Rates*
Subsequent to Adequate Irradiation Used Postoperatively or Alone

| Survival Over | Length of Survival | | | Quality of Survival | | |
| | Total Possible | No. of Survivors | Per Cent of Survivals | Percentile Recovery Grade** | | |
				I	II	III
5 Years	564	196	35%	80%	15%	5%
10 ″	412	106	26	82	16	2
15 ″	258	51	20	84	14	2
20 ″	111	21	19	90	10	—

* From patients adequately irradiated, 83.2% postoperatively, 1939–58. Follow-up complete to 1964.

** Grading of Recovery: Grade I —Good—Active useful life
Grade II —Fair —Partial disability
Grade III—Poor —Total disability:
physical and/or mental.

content, we have recently reviewed and re-assessed the degree of recovery at the end of every 5-year period in the case of each patient who has survived more than 5 years.

Among our patients whose brain and other intracranial tissues were exposed to intensive irradiation more than 5, 10, 15 or 20 years ago, the overall proportion of long-term survivals and good recoveries is higher than most physicians would dare to predict (Table 2). The longer the survival, the higher the proportion of good recovery among the survivors. It is significant that only 11 or 5.5 per cent of the 196 patients who have survived over 5 years were totally disabled 5 years after irradiation. The rate of total disability is only 2 per cent among the 10- and 15-year survivors, whereas it is nil in the group of 21 who have survived more than 20 years following radiation therapy of adequate intensity.

Results of Treatment by Irradiation Only. The overall results of adequate treatment with irradiation alone in the management of primary intracranial neoplasms deserve to be reviewed with particular attention, since there is very scanty information in that respect in the current medical literature. Of the 564 primary intracranial neoplasms that we have irradiated more than 5 years ago, a total of 95 patients (80 with gliomata and 15 with non-gliomatous tumors) had no surgical removal of their tumor and were treated only with radiation. In regard to the life expectancy of patients so treated, the long-term survival and recovery rates subsequent to the treatment with irradiation alone of 95 primary intracranial neoplasms of different types have been tabulated side by side (Table 3).

It is shown in Table 3 that 95 of our patients were treated with radiation alone more than 5 years ago; 59, over 10 years ago; 30, over 15 years ago; and 13, over 20 years ago. The percentages of those who have survived more than 5, 10 and 15 years after irradiation are practically equal after each period of time as they rate 36 and 37 per cent, whereas the rate is 23

TABLE 3. Primary Intracranial Neoplasms
Long-Term Survival and Recovery Rates*
Subsequent to Treatment with Adequate Irradiation Alone

Survival Over	Total Possible	No. of Survivors	Per Cent of Survivals	Quality of Survival Percentile Recovery Grade**		
	Length of Survival			I	II	III
5 Years	95	34	36%	85%	6%	9%
10 "	59	22	37	95	—	5
15 "	30	11	37	100	—	—
20 "	13	3	23	100	—	—

* From 80 gliomata and 15 non-gliomatous tumors treated without surgical removal, a total of 95 or 16.8% of all primary intracranial tumors adequately irradiated, 1939–58. Follow-up complete to 1964.

** Grading of Recovery: Grade I —Good—Active useful life
Grade II —Fair —Partial disability
Grade III—Poor —Total disability:
physical and/or mental.

per cent for those who have lived more than 20 years following the onset of irradiation. The actual degree of recovery at 5 and 10 years has been quite good when considering that only 3 of the 34 survivors or 9 per cent of the patients treated with irradiation alone were totally disabled at 5 years, and only one or 5 per cent of the 22 survivors at 10 years was totally incapacitated. The 11 patients who survived over 15 years, and among them the 3 who were alive over 20 years after irradiation were all in perfect condition.

The long-term survival and recovery rates subsequent to the treatment of primary intracranial neoplasms with adequate irradiation alone may be considered statistically as not significant because of the relatively small number of patients so treated. These rates at least indicate a strong trend as to the kind of results which may be anticipated whenever larger groups of patients will become available for long-term assessment.

Influence of Decompressive Procedures Over Long-Term Results. In the immediate management of patients treated for inoperable intracranial tumors, decompressive measures, in our opinion, been most useful during and after their course of irradiation. In several cases dramatic improvement of patients' condition has been observed soon after the shunt had been established, even before irradiation was initiated. Shunts have the advantage of being relatively simple procedures and seem to be particularly indicated in the management of tumors located in a region from which they can rarely be extirpated as in the mid-brain area and to a lesser extent in the brain stem. Shunts are sometimes useful in the management of medulloblastomas located in the posterior fossa.

The various surgical procedures used for relieving increased intracranial pressure must have influenced the length of survival in some cases just as much as the radiation therapy administered. From the 80 patients whose gliomas were directly treated with radiation only 24 patients had some type of surgical decompression without surgical extirpation, and 11 of these survived 5 years or longer. Various types of shunts were the mode of decompression in 9 of those 11 survivors.

In the non-gliomatous tumors, decompression was needed prior to irradiation in 7 of 15 cases, but it was not in the remaining 8 patients who had presented no significant evidence of increased intracranial pressure before they were irradiated for cerebral vascular tumors.

Follow-up Special Procedures for Evaluation of Treatment Results

In the evaluation of results of treatment, the methods which are currently utilized for the investigation and diagnosis of primary intracranial neoplasms are not generally used. It is customary to rely upon clinical results almost exclusively. Air studies subsequent to completion of treatment, either immediately after a course of radiation therapy or perhaps a few months later, have been performed occasionally. Follow-up pneumo-encephalography was accomplished in not less than 8 of our own cases for patients who had been treated by irradiation alone mostly in medulloblastomas (Figs. 7, 8, 9 and 10) and a few sarcomas.

The general opinion is that follow-up special procedures are not really essential to a patient's welfare, even though it may seem desirable from the academic standpoint. The use of cerebral angiography for the same purposes has limited applications for the same reasons. The actual value of post-treatment gamma encephalography is questionable when dealing with patients previously subjected to surgical removal with or without post-operative irradiation. However, this is a relatively simple test to perform and, when a preoperative scan has been positive, it should prove a useful procedure in the assessment of results following treatment with irradiation alone. Post-treatment echo-encephalography, thermographic scans and electro-encephalography are considered of limited scope as methods of evaluation of radiation effects in the treatment of intracranial neoplasms.

Our results in the treatment of primary intracranial neoplasms have been presented for all cases in which irradiation was used either as a postoperative procedure in combination with surgical removal of tumors or else as the sole method of active control over the neoplastic process. Those results are complete and valid, inasmuch as the length and quality of survivals have been estimated globally. In subsequent chapters the role of radiation therapy in the management of gliomatous and non-gliomatous tumors will be evaluated separately and more fully for each category of tumor.

Effects of Irradiation in Treatment of Intracranial Gliomas— Treatment Results by Histologic Groups

EVALUATION of the effects of adequate irradiation in the treatment of primary intracranial gliomas is presented here primarily on a statistical basis. Considerable data have been derived from the accumulated clinical observations recorded over years of careful and continuous follow-up of every patient that we have adequately irradiated in the treatment of brain tumors. The experience and results of many workers have been reviewed and reported in order to complete, in relation to the methods of treatment, an overall appraisal which may be essentially objective.

Surgical management of intracranial gliomata dominates the scene in the final diagnosis and initial treatment. Results of surgical treatment alone, however, indicate that the majority of intracranial gliomata cannot be extirpated completely and reactivate sooner than later. Postoperative radiation therapy adequately administered seems to have considerable therapeutic efficacy in medulloblastomas, less in other gliomas, perhaps none in some. In the management of certain gliomata, we have used intensive adequate irradiation as the sole therapeutic agent with some degree of efficacy. The clinical course of patients untreated for intracranial gliomas is generally known as unfavorable, but well-documented series suitable for comparison with the outcome of treated patients are not commonly available.

It is not intended to present here a plea for or against any particular method of treatment. Unquestionably, surgical procedures are of paramount importance and play the most important role in the management of intracranial gliomata (see page 56). Irradiation has a definite therapeutic value. I do register the plea that irradiation when and where indicated be adequate. Adequate irradiation means that the plan of treatment must not consist of some magic formula or standard prescription applicable to all cases of a certain type of glioma. Irradiation may be adequate when the plan of treatment takes into account the characteristics of respective tumor entities and other important general considerations outlined in previous chapters. Radiation therapy is adequate when the total dose absorbed by a tumor over a certain period of time is such that the intensity of irradiation is high enough to induce maximum growth restraint and regression, without exceeding the tolerance of adjacent brain tissue and normal intervening structures. This must be accomplished without overlooking the importance of the total volume of tissue exposed to such intensive irradiation during the overall therapeutic process. Under these circumstances, it is easy to conceive why there are no great variations in relation to the tumor doses recommended subsequently for the irradiation of different gliomas.

Since the nomenclature of gliomatous tumors is often confusing, synonymous or equivalent terminology will be indicated as the occasion may arise.

Considering that primary intracranial gliomas arise from three groups of cells: the astrocytes, the oligodendrocytes, and the ependymal cells, and in view also of the fact that the cellular variety giving rise to medulloblastomas is disputed by neuropathologists, the gliomas will be studied in four groups:

1) Gliomas of astrocytic origin;
2) Gliomas of oligodendrocytic origin;
3) Gliomas of ependymal cell origin;
4) Medulloblastomas.

LIFE EXPECTANCY OF PATIENTS WITH GLIOMAS

In the course of management of patients with intracranial neoplasms, the referring specialist, the family physician, the relatives and others often inquire as to the life expectancy of patients subjected to intensive radiation therapy as part or all of their treatment for a particular type of brain tumor. Considering the number and variety of cases of intracranial neoplasms that we have treated with ionizing radiation from 1939 to 1958 inclusive, we have attempted to provide a reasonable answer to such a type of query by preparing life expectancy tables. For that purpose, primary intracranial gliomata have been separated from the non-gliomatous intracranial tumors and assembled by histological groups, and also by anatomic location when tumors are affecting the mid-brain and brain stem.

Life Expectancy (1 to 20 years) with Gliomas of Different Types Treated by Surgical Removal plus Irradiation and by Irradiation Alone

A life expectancy table has been prepared for all patients treated for intracranial gliomata either by surgical removal followed by irradiation or solely by irradiation (Table 4). This is based upon the actual survival rates of 494 patients treated more than 5 years ago. Of the 494 gliomata, 367

TABLE 4. Primary Intracranial Gliomata
Life Expectancy of Patients Treated by
Surgical Removal and Irradiation or Irradiation Alone

Type or Location of Glioma	Percentile Life Expectancy Greater Than					
	1 Year	3 Years	5 Years	10 Years	15 Years	20 Years
Glioblastoma	44	13	7	4	2	0
Glioma—unclassified	71	48	30	20	13	13
Astrocytoma	86	65	52	31	24	21
Oligodendroglioma-blastoma	100	79	50	33	18	15
Ependymoma-blastoma	90	75	70	56	52	43
Medulloblastoma	74	36	27	17	9	8
Mid-brain tumors	70	54	46	39	30	20
Brain stem tumors	56	29	29	24	23	20
Average Rates:	66	40	30	20	15	15

Table drawn up from actual survival rates of 494 patients irradiated adequately, 1939 to 1958 inclusive. Clinical follow-up complete to 1964, ranging from a minimum of 5 years up to 25 years. Of the 494 patients, 367 were treated over 10 years ago; 229, over 15 years; and 99, over 20 years. Surgical removal plus postoperative irradiation: 414 gliomata or 83.8%.—Irradiation alone: 80 or 16.2%.

were treated over 10 years ago; 229, over 15 years ago; and 99, over 20 years ago. Our clinical follow-up is complete to 1964, so that it ranges from a minimum of 5 years up to 25 after irradiation. The tabulation of life expectancy shows the percentage of survivors who, in each type of glioma, have survived over 1, 3, 5, 10, 15, and 20 years after irradiation. In 414 (83.8 per cent) of our intracranial gliomata, irradiation was used postoperatively, whereas it was the sole treatment in the 80 other cases.

At one glance (Table 4), it is obvious that the lowest survival rates are in glioblastomas, which account for nearly one third of the entire group of gliomata in the present series. Actually, if glioblastomas were excluded, the overall average 5-year survival rate for the rest of the glioma group would be approximately 40 per cent instead of the overall 30 per cent appearing on Table 4. At the same time the average survival rates over 10, 15 and 20 years would rise proportionately. The highest survival rates are in the group of gliomas arising from ependymal cells, but these represent a relatively small group or 4 per cent only of our entire series of gliomata. The life expectancy of patients irradiated adequately in the treatment of medulloblastomas appears to be more favorable than generally recognized, with 27 per cent 5-year and 17 per cent 10-year survival rates. In mid-brain and brain stem tumors, overall long-term survival rates are substantially superior to those generally expected for gliomas located in such critical areas.

Life Expectancy (1 to 20 years) with Gliomas of Different Types Treated Solely by Irradiation

The life expectancy of patients treated with irradiation alone for a variety of intracranial gliomata, either grouped by histologic types or according to their particular anatomic location, is not presented on a percentile basis in Table 5. Accordingly, Table 5 has been drawn up to show in each category of tumor treated with radiation only, the actual proportion of survivors over the total number of patients treated, that proportion of survivals appearing over 1, 3, 5, 10, 15 and 20 years following irradiation.

Of our 80 cases of gliomata treated with radiation alone (Table 5), 11

TABLE 5. Life Expectancy of Patients Treated with Irradiation Alone*
In Primary Intracranial Neoplasms

Gliomata (80 cases)		Proportion of Survivals Over				
	1 Year	3 Years	5 Years	10 Years	15 Years	20 Years
Glioblastoma	2/5	1/5	0/5	—	—	—
Glioma—unclassified	2/3	1/3	0/3	0/1	0/1	0/1
Astrocytoma	2/3	0/3	0/3	0/1	—	—
Medulloblastoma	8/10	4/10	4/10	2/7	1/4	0/1
Mid-brain	20/29	15/29	12/29	7/17	1/5	0/2
Brain stem	15/30	8/30	8/30	5/20	4/12	1/5
All Types	49/80	29/80	24/80	14/46	6/22	1/9
Average Rates	61%	36%	30%	30%	27%	11%
Non-gliomatous Tumors (15 cases)	14/15	13/15	10/15	8/13	5/8	2/4

* Table drawn up by showing the actual proportion of survivors over the total number of patients who, by the end of each period of time indicated above, had been treated only with radiation—a total of 95 patients from 1939 to 1958 inclusive.

Clinical follow-up complete to 1964, ranging from a minimum of 5 years up to 25.

consisted of tumors derived from astrocytes (5 glioblastomas, 3 unclassified gliomas and 3 astrocytomas). It must be noted that only 2 of these have survived over 3 years and not 1 over 5 years or longer. Only 2 of those 11 patients might have survived over 10 years. Each of the 11 patients was in critical condition, having large gliomas considered inoperable on account of their location in the cerebral motor cortex and probable ensuing marked disability had they survived operation. Among the patients treated with irradiation alone, 10 had medulloblastomas proven by aspiration biopsy. The majority of cases (59 of 80) were mid-brain and brain stem tumors which deserve to be discussed in a separate chapter.

Expectancy for Good Recovery in All Types of Intracranial Gliomas

In all types of gliomas, the expectancy for a good or fair recovery may rise very high in relation with the duration of survival, whether short or long. Among the 150 5-year survivors in the group of gliomas treated by irradiation, either postoperatively or alone, only 6.6 per cent were totally disabled at the end of the 5-year period Of the 10 patients who showed a poor recovery at 5 years, 7 had been treated for astrocytomas, 2 for mid-brain and 1 for pontine tumors.

GLIOMAS OF ASTROCYTIC ORIGIN

Approximately 75 per cent of all intracranial gliomas are comprising malignant tumors originating from astrocytes. Truly comparable cases must be grouped together inasmuch as possible for presentation of a reliable analysis of treatment results. These may differ from one series of cases to another depending upon the relative degree of histologic differentiation or grading used as index of the degree of malignancy of tumors. Results must be compared also in relation to the method of treatment applied. Considering the above criteria, the results of treatment of astrocytic tumors will be assessed under three groups: glioblastoma multiforme, representing approximately 50 per cent of the total, unclassified gliomas (10 per cent) and low-grade astrocytomas (40 per cent).

Our total series of gliomas of astrocytic origin comprises 339 cases. For those using Kernohan's classification[55], these cases would represent all astrocytomas classified as Grade I, II, III and IV grouped together. All but 11 patients were treated by surgical removal and adequate postoperative irradiation. The overall survival rates have been estimated at 62.5 per cent over 1 year, 36 per cent over 3 years, and 27 per cent over 5 years. Over 10, 15 and 20 years, because of the sharp disappearance of patients treated for glioblastomas, the survival rates have levelled off to an average of 11 per cent. In the analysis of long-term results, it seems preferable to group astrocytic tumors according to the pathological grading which, in our own material, corresponds to glioblastoma multiforme, unclassified gliomas, and low-grade astrocytomas of the common variety.

Glioblastoma Multiforme

Irrespective of its location in the central nervous system, glioblastoma multiforme (classified in other terminology as: spongioblastoma multiforme or astrocytoma Grade III to IV) is universally recognized as the most malignant type of glioma. Its incidence is the highest of all malignant gliomata in nearly every large series of cases. In our own material, 40 per cent of 449 histologically proven gliomata have been diagnosed glioblastoma multiforme. This histologic variety of glioma is found predominantly in males, between 30 to 50 years of age, mostly in the cerebral hemispheres. Judging from the duration of symptoms prior to diagnosis it is usually a fast growing tumor. Fraenkel and German[35] have reported an average duration of symptoms of less than 6 months prior to diagnosis in 70 per cent of 219 cases, and of more than 1 year in only 17 per cent. The immediate prognosis is very poor if untreated. Bailey[8] suggested 15 months as a probable maximum life expectancy.

Following craniotomy and surgical removal of the tumor, Elvidge, Penfield and Cone[31] have reported an average survival of 8.5 months in 22 cases. MacCarty[72] has treated by surgical removal alone 60 patients with glioblastoma multiforme. Only 2 of his 60 patients have survived over 5 years, a rate of 3.4 per cent as compared with 7 per cent in our series of 171 patients treated by a combination of surgical removal and postoperative irradiation.

In 183 cases treated surgically, Fraenkel and German[35] have reported an average postoperative survival period of 3 months. Only 13 per cent of their patients have survived over 1 year following surgical treatment. These included 21 patients who received doses of radiation therapy that can be considered adequate at least at the higher levels. In their comparison of 21 patients who were irradiated postoperatively (2700 to 5900 r, tumor dose) within 60 days after operation, the results during the first 12 months showed a greater percentage of survivors in the irradiated group. The length of survival appeared to be related in some degree to the size of the tumor dose, and they reported that those who survived over 9 months had received 4000 rads or more. Regarding the degree of postoperative recovery, only 40 per cent of their patients showed either slight postoperative disability or none. The extent of surgical management consisted of biopsy only in 25 cases, partial extirpation in 105, and radical removal in the remainder of the cases.

Of the 176 patients that we irradiated with kilovoltage X-radiation in the management of their glioblastoma multiforme, 171 were irradiated postoperatively and 5 were treated solely with radiation. Both the short and long-term results have confirmed that life expectancy in glioblastomas remains low despite intensive postoperative irradiation. The overall results (Table 4) suggest that adequate radiation therapy following surgical removal must be useful, since 44 per cent of our 176 patients have survived over 1 year. This is contrasting with 13 per cent for the 183 patients of Fraenkel and German who treated these almost exclusively by surgical procedures. Their longest survival was 48 months, whereas 7 per cent or 13 of our patients who had intensive postoperative irradiation have survived over 5 years.

The quality of recovery among the patients that we have irradiated for a part of their treatment was graded as good, with return to normal life for most of the duration of their survival in 75 per cent of those who survived less than 5 years. In the 13 patients who have survived over 5 years, the degree of recovery was such that 10 have been in excellent condition, 3 have remained with partial disability, and not a single patient has been totally disabled.

Using megavoltage (1,000,000 volt x-rays), Jones[49] reported on 33 patients treated for glioblastoma from 1937 to 1953. In his opinion, a proportion of tumors are moderately radiosensitive in the glioblastoma multiforme group but the response is usually transient. The lack of radiosensitivity of glioblastomas as compared with that of the normal brain is the essential difficulty.

With 23 Mev X-radiation, Arnold, Bailey, Harvey and Hass[3] have reported on the treatment of 9 glioblastomas in which they used tumor doses varying from 5500 to 6500 r in 17 to 30 days up to 7500 r in 26 to 30 days. They expressed the opinion that, with such quality of radiation, well-defined homogeneous beams permit more precise localization, more uniform dose distribution and minimal irradiation of adjacent healthy tissues. Of the 9 patients so treated, 5 have enjoyed a useful survival for 14 to 21 months. Histopathologic studies made subsequently revealed more intense changes than usually observed following kilovoltage x-ray therapy.

Treatment solely by irradiation has not been common practice in the management of glioblastoma multiforme. Our experience is limited to 5 cases. The diagnosis had been established by needle biopsy. As shown in Table 5, only 2 of our 5 patients have survived over 1 year, one of these having exceeded 3 years. Not enough cases have been treated with radiation alone to determine its relative value, even less to allow for comparison with other methods of treatment.

The potential role of chemotherapy is still under investigation. Llewellyn and Creech[69] have perfused with various chemotherapeutic agents 24 adult patients. The diagnosis of glioblastoma multiforme had been established by histopathological studies. In 18 cases, thio-tepa was used. Llewellyn et al. expressed the opinion that tumors are not eradicated by perfusion with the chemotherapeutic agents presently available and that life is not prolonged.

After reviewing and comparing the results of treatment by various methods, we are convinced that the treatment of choice of glioblastoma multiforme should consist primarily of surgical decompression and removal followed with intensive irradiation. Clinical results suggest that good palliation of symptoms and appreciable growth restraint can be accomplished. Survival rates indicate that life may be prolonged by some months for the majority of patients and exceptionally for a few years. A high degree of immediate recovery may be anticipated in most cases and for the greater part of the duration of survival.

The extent of surgical extirpation should be such as to provide a good decompression by removing the bulk of the tumor and thus reduce the volume of tissue whose neoplastic activity may be controlled by subsequent irradiation. Such surgical removal is justifiable inasmuch as it can be performed with minimum risk for the patient. That is particularly important when a tumor is located in the motor area of the dominant hemisphere, as patients may then remain with serious deficit of normal functions.

Adequate irradiation can be accomplished with kilovoltage X-radiation, but megavoltage is preferable although the results may not necessarily be better when the latter is being used. Protraction of dose is most important.

In irradiation of glioblastoma multiforme, the optimum time-dose relation would seem to be of the order of 6500 rads tumor dose, over periods of approximately 50 to 60 days, using Cobalt[60] radiation.

Unclassified Gliomata

These primary brain tumors represent a group of malignant gliomata that neuropathologists ordinarily find difficult to classify either in the glioblastoma or else in the low-grade astrocytoma groups, or even in other groups of tumors of glial origin. Unclassified gliomas are mixed tumors which histologically show a mixture of a variety of glial cells so dispersed within the tumor that no predominant pattern is distinguishable. In the simplified classification of gliomata that Ringert[100] proposed, such cases would be classified in the "intermediate group". In Kernohan's classification[55] these seem to correspond to astrocytomas Grade II to III. Other equivalent appellations are astroblastoma and spongioblastoma polare.

There are 40 unclassified gliomas in our series of 494 intracranial gliomata. Of 40 patients, 37 have been treated with craniotomy, decompression and surgical removal followed by irradiation (Table 4), whereas 3 have been treated with irradiation alone (Table 5). It is difficult to find pure surgical series suitable for comparison of treatment results of unclassified gliomas in relation to other methods of treatment, whether this was by surgical removal combined with postoperative irradiation or solely by irradiation. One cannot be too certain of comparing treatment results in identical histologic tumors. Considerable variation in terminology exists and reflects wide individual differences of interpretation among pathologists when they classify tumors in this intermediate group between the highly malignant glioblastoma multiforme and the less malignant astrocytoma. Results reveal (Table 4) that both short and long-term survivals are better in unclassified gliomata than in glioblastomas, but are not as good as in the ordinary or low-grade astrocytomas.

Long-term recovery rates have been remarkably good, since only 1 of 12 5-year survivors was living with partial disability at 5 years, and not 1 was totally disabled among those who have survived over 5, 10, 15 or 20 years after treatment.

Because of the moderately malignant character of most unclassified gliomata and their natural tendency to be infiltrating in type, our aim is to irradiate postoperatively up to an average tumor dose of 6000 rads over a period of 50 to 60 days, using megavoltage with Cobalt[60] radiation.

Astrocytoma

This category of gliomas is grouping tumors which are relatively well differentiated histologically and can be readily identified as being of astrocytic origin. These gliomas are often designated as the common variety of astrocytomas. In Kernohan's classification they correspond to astrocytomas Grade I to II. The term astroblastoma is now rarely used by neuropathologists to classify low-grade and slowly growing astrocytomas in which some astroblasts are present. Bailey and Cushing[7] have divided astrocytomas into the fibrous and protoplasmic varieties. Elvidge, Penfield and Cone[31] have suggested that astrocytomas be divided into three subgroups: piloid, diffuse and gemistocytic.

Intracranial astrocytomas involve the cerebral hemispheres in about 65 to 75 per cent of the cases and the cerebellum in 20 to 25 per cent. They may be found in the mid-brain, brain stem or pons, and occasionally in the optic chiasm and nerves. Our series comprises 123 intracranial astrocytomas of the common or well differentiated variety (Grade I to II). These include 3 tumors which shall be discussed with the gliomas arising from the optic chiasm and nerves under separate heading at the end of this section of the present chapter. Astrocytomas involving the mid-brain (7 cases) or the pons (2 cases) are not included among the 123 astrocytic tumors under review at present. Such tumors will be considered separately from the majority of intracranial gliomata of astrocytic origin. They shall be grouped with other tumors located in the same critical areas, where the hazard to the patient's life is more relative to the location of the new growth than to its histopathology.

Levy and Elvidge[67] have reviewed 165 intracranial astrocytomas treated between 1940 and 1949 at the Montreal Neurological Institute. Of their 165 astrocytomas, 73 per cent were supratentorial and 27 per cent infratentorial. Supratentorial astrocytomas involving the cerebral hemispheres were subclassified into piloid, gemistocytic and diffuse types which have been analyzed in subgroups. All cerebellar astrocytomas were classed in the piloid type. Astrocytomas involving the third ventricle, pons, and optic nerves were also of the piloid variety, but have been studied in separate subgroups according to their respective anatomic location instead of by histologic diagnosis.

The prognosis of intracranial astrocytomas varies markedly with the anatomic location, whether the tumor is supratentorial in the cerebrum or infratentorial in the cerebellum. The role of postoperative radiation therapy also varies in that respect.

Supratentorial Astrocytomas

Astrocytomas located above the tentorium and arising from the cerebral hemispheres represent the largest group of cerebral gliomata after glioblastoma multiforme. The majority of astrocytomas involve the frontal lobes, and many in that region have been found to have crossed the midline to the other side (in 10 per cent of 53 piloid astrocytomas reported by Levy and

Elvidge[67] (See Plate 2). The diffuse type is observed predominantly in the temporal region. Most of the cerebral astrocytomas are slowly growing. The average duration prior to diagnosis and treatment seems to vary from 2 to 4 years and even longer, with the result that tumors in that category are often sizable when discovered.

In cerebral astrocytomas, surgical treatment consisting of craniotomy is indicated primarily to accomplish decompression and obtain tissue for histologic diagnosis, and then to remove the bulk of the tumor if not all of it. However, it seems that surgical extirpation in toto may be feasible in approximately one third of the cases only. According to Levy and Elvidge[67], the fact that the removal of an astrocytoma is known to be incomplete does not necessarily indicate a poor prognosis, but merely that it was difficult for the surgeon to determine the limits of the tumor at the time of operation.

The series of astrocytomas reviewed by Levy and Elvidge comprises 113 supratentorial tumors of which 87 were available for study of post operative results once operative deaths had been excluded. Of those 87 patients, we have counted 42 who were treated by surgery only and 45 who had surgical removal followed with irradiation. Since both groups are practically identical in number, a close comparison of treatment results is possible between the two groups (Table 6). Survival rates are presented over

TABLE 6.   Cerebral Astrocytomas***
Five-Year Survival Rates in Patients Treated by
Surgical Removal Alone or Postoperative Irradiation

	Surgical Removal Alone* (42 cases)		Postoperative Irradiation* (45 cases)		Postoperative Irradiation** (105 cases)	
Survival Over	No. of Survivors	Per Cent	No. of Survivors	Per Cent	No. of Survivors	Per Cent
1 Year	34	81%	37	82%	90	86%
3 Years	22	52	28	62	67	64
5 Years	11	26	16	36	51	49

* Table prepared from analysis of data presented by Levy and Elvidge in study of 87 patients followed up after surgical treatment—42 of these had surgery only—and 45 had postoperative irradiation.

** Author's series, comprising 105 patients irradiated postoperatively from 1939 to 1958 and including the 45 cases reported by Levy and Elvidge. Follow-up complete to 1964.

*** All three series above include supratentorial astrocytomas (Grade I and II) involving cerebral hemispheres only. Mid-brain and pontine astrocytomas have been excluded.

1, 3, and 5 years following surgical removal, 29 complete and 58 incomplete. In view of the fact that tumor extirpation was considered incomplete in 58 cases of cerebral astrocytomas and that postoperative irradiation was used in 45 cases only, it is obvious that the group of 42 patients treated by surgery only comprises 13 incomplete removals not exposed to radiation.

The proportion of those who survived over the first year following surgical treatment, whether alone or with irradiation, is practically identical in each group. At the end of the 3- and 5-year periods, survival rates are higher by 10 per cent among patients adequately irradiated, nearly all on account of incomplete removal. Further analysis of cases disclosed that approximately two thirds of those who had had a surgical removal considered complete and accordingly had received no postoperative irradiation failed to survive over 5 years and died of their astrocytomas. From those observations it will appear subsequently that survival rates following surgical removal only (complete in 29 and incomplete in 13 cases) have not been as favorable in cerebral astrocytomas as they have been in the cerebellar group.

The author's series (Table 6) comprises 105 astrocytomas involving cerebral hemispheres only, so that it can be compared with other series, such as those made out from Levy and Elvidge's cases. It must be mentioned here that this series of ours happens to include the 45 patients (Table 6) irradiated postoperatively in the treatment of the hemispheral cerebral astrocytomas reported among Levy and Elvidge's cases. Mid-brain and pontine astrocytomas have been excluded from all three survival series shown on Table 6. It appears in that Table that 49 per cent of our 105 patients irradiated for hemispheral astrocytomas have survived over 5 years. It should be added that 18 of 83, or 22 per cent, have survived over 10 years, that 7 of 40 or 18 percent have survived over 15 years, and that 2 of 19 or 11 per cent have survived over 20 years.

In evaluating the results of operation for intracranial gliomas, Mac-Carty[72] has reported a 5-year survival rate of 43.8 per cent of a group of 16 traced patients who had hemispheral astrocytomas (Grades I and II) removed surgically. Horrax[45] called attention to certain favorable types of brain tumors, when he reviewed some 1718 verified intracranial tumors in which there were 314 cases of cerebral astrocytomas. In his opinion, approximately 10 per cent of cerebral astrocytomas can be regarded as benign and favorable because these are cystic and so well demarcated tumors that extirpation in toto is feasible: of 32 patients in that category who had lived 5 years or longer, 21 had a useful life from 5 to 17 years after surgical removal, a good recovery rate of 65.6 per cent.

From the data presented by Levy and Elvidge[67] on astrocytomas involving the cerebral hemispheres it is estimated that, following surgical removal alone, 26 per cent of 42 of their patients have survived over 5 years. In another group of their series, 36 per cent of 45 patients have survived over 5 years following treatment by surgery and irradiation. These 45 cases are included in the author's series of 105 patients (Table 6) whom we have irradiated more than 5 years ago, following surgical removal of astrocytomas located in the cerebral hemispheres exclusively. Of the 105 patients, 51 or 49 per cent have survived over 5 years.

According to Levy and Elvidge, the length of survival is greater after surgery and roentgen-ray therapy than after surgery alone in the piloid and diffuse types of astrocytomas involving cerebral hemispheres. They observed the opposite in the gemistocytic variety which in their series represented 28.5 per cent of the cases assessed in that respect. The percentage of 5-year survivals was higher in the first two histologic varieties and lesser in the third. The overall 5-year survival rate for all patients exposed to postoperative irradiation in their series turned out to be 10 per cent higher than in the non-irradiated. They have observed relatively the same difference in survival rates between tumors completely and incompletely eradicated at operation. The latter observation may be significant in view of the fact that cerebral astrocytomas are by far the tumors most commonly exposed to postoperative irradiation.

From the standpoint of longevity, all the evidence presented above seems to indicate that patients irradiated postoperatively for supratentorial astrocytomas involving cerebral hemispheres may be expected to do better than those treated by surgical removal only. Five-year results after surgical removal alone have been superior in the treatment of benign cystic cerebral astrocytomas as reported by Horrax, but these represent a relatively small porportion (approximately 10 per cent) of all cerebral hemispheral astrocytomas.

Clinically, subjective and objective improvement has been observed in the majority of patients who survived operation following surgical decompression and tumor extirpation, including partial lobectomy of frontal, temporal or even occipital lobes. Several patients have made a slow immediate recovery and were not in good condition when postoperative irradiation was initiated within a couple of weeks after operation. By the time that adequate irradiation has been completed most patients usually have made a satisfactory recovery. The maximum degree of recovery may not be fully appreciable for 3 to 6 and possibly up to 12 months after completion of treatment.

On a long-term basis, the lowest rate of complete recovery of all our clinical material has been found in the group of patients treated for cerebral astrocytomas. This is true in relation to every group of patients that we have irradiated and followed up for various types of primary intracranial gliomata. Actually, 60 to 65 per cent of the patients among our 5-, 10-, 15-, and 20-year survivors have made a Grade I recovery and remained perfectly well following surgical removal and irradiation of their hemispheral astrocytomas. The corollary is that the proportion of 5- and 10-year survivors with disability, partial in 23 per cent and total in 12 per cent, is higher than in any other group of patients that we have treated for intracranial tumors and reviewed for evaluation of the quality of survival.

The lower rates of full recovery among patients treated for cerebral astrocytomas are probably attributable to factors other than irradiation. Recovery rates following surgical treatment alone are difficult to find for comparison purposes, although the literature is full of references to useful survivals. These would appear to be approximately the same as when radiation therapy has been added to the treatment.

There is no appreciable evidence that our recovery rates may have been affected adversely by adequate intensive irradiation administered postoperatively. Persistent neurologic signs and partial disability in some of the patients not irradiated after operation suggest that some of the brain damage caused directly or indirectly by the tumor itself has not been corrected by the methods of treatment used in those cases to remove tumor tissue or restrain its growth. The proximity of tumors to the motor area or their interference with visual centers and fiber tracts seem to be major factors in preventing full recovery in some of the patients.

Technically, we presently treat cerebral astrocytomas postoperatively with Cobalt [60] high energy radiation by delivering tumor doses averaging 5000 to 6000 rads over a period of 45 to 50 days, and perhaps slightly higher doses in the treatment of recurrences.

Radiation therapy alone has not been used extensively enough (3 cases only) by the author, or others to my knowledge, to warrant any conclusion. Chemotherapeutic agents remain practically untried in astrocytomas.

The evidence presented above strongly indicates that supratentorial astrocytomas arising from the cerebral hemispheres can be treated best by surgical removal combined with postoperative irradiation. Comparative survival rates strongly suggest that beyond the third year after treatment, longevity is increasingly greater among patients who had postoperative irradiation than in those treated solely by surgery. The rates of full and lasting recovery (60 to 65 per cent) are satisfactory but may be improved. This might be accomplished through less radical surgical extirpation of tumor and greater reliance upon adequate radiation therapy. The value of adequate irradiation, administered postoperatively, is unquestionable in the management of cerebral hemispheral astrocytomas.

Treatment of Recurrent Cerebral Astrocytomas

Radiation therapy may be used advantageously in the management of patients with *recurrences* of cerebral astrocytomas. Our series of 105 cases of hemispheral cerebral astrocytomas comprises 12 patients who were irradiated for tumor recurrences. Initially 9 of these 12 patients were treated by surgery alone. These had radiation therapy only later after their tumor had recurred. Intervals between surgical treatment and recurrences varied from 30 months to 5 years in 5 cases, were of 9 years in 2 and 18 years in 1. Tumor recurred 7 months only after operation in the remaining case. Five of the 9 patients treated for postoperative recurrences had radiation therapy only. Four had a second operation before irradiation was used.

All 5 patients, irradiated only at the time of recurrence of their cerebral astrocytomas, have improved clinically during and after treatment. One patient made a complete recovery and is alive and well at the age of 64, 14 years after the onset of irradiation. A woman, who had developed post-operative recurrence of her tumor some 2½ years after surgical removal solely, recovered under irradiation and remained symtom-free over 3 years, after which she gradually became disabled but was still capable of reading and caring for herself until the last months of her 64-month survival. Another patient survived 9 years following irradiation administered to control his recurrent tumor, but the quality of his survival was good over a period of 1½ years only, and then he began to deteriorate slowly until he became totally disabled physically and mentally. The remaining 2 patients had brief periods of partial recovery and died 8 and 11 months respectively from the onset of belated radiation therapy. Only 1 of the 5 patients had a survival shorter than the interval between his previous operation and the time of irradiation for recurrence.

Four patients, whose cerebral astrocytomas reactivated following surgical treatment alone, were subjected to a second craniotomy and subsequently to radiation therapy. Two of these were irradiated soon after their second operation. A woman, who had developed recurrence 5 years after initial surgical removal, survived nearly 12 more years after further surgery plus irradiation; although she remained partially disabled, she was relatively well at the 5- and 10-year periods of her survival as estimated from the time of irradiation. The second patient improved and made partial recovery for 15 months before gradually deteriorating mentally and physically until he died exactly 5 years after the onset of postoperative irradiation. The other 2 patients received radiation therapy 2 years following their second craniotomy when their tumors reactivated once more. Both improved clinically as they made satisfactory partial recoveries which lasted approximately 1 year in each case before deteriorating and expiring respectively 18 and 34 months following onset of irradiation.

When cerebral astrocytomas have recurred subsequent to previous combined treatment with surgical extirpation and intensive postoperative irradiation, further remission of symptoms and perhaps prolongation of life might be accomplished. When a second course of intensive radiation therapy is administered, there is a potential risk of postradiation necrosis, should the patient survive long enough. Two cases of cerebral astrocytomas exposed to a second course of intensive irradiation, because of recurrence, have clinically recovered and remained reasonably well for the major part of their respective survivals of 1 and 4 years. A third patient failed to improve following a further course of radiation therapy and died 3 months later.

In the treatment of 3 other cases of post operative and postradiation recurrences, a second surgical removal was the sole selected therapeutic procedure; 2 patients improved temporarily and survived 2 and 3 years respectively, whereas the third died at operation.

Recurrent cerebral astrocytomas are currently treated with megavoltage, using Cobalt[60] radiation, and tumor doses averaging 5000 to 6000 rads over a period of 45 to 50 days and sometimes 60 days if the volume of tissue to be irradiated is rather large. Occasionally the total tumor dose is brought up to a maximum of 6500 rads.

Infratentorial Astrocytomas

Astrocytic gliomata located in the posterior fossa consist almost exclusively of cerebellar tumors found in children, adolescents and few young adults. The average age incidence of infratentorial astrocytomas ranges from 12 to 15 years. Our youngest patient was 26 months old. Cerebellar astrocytomas are seen more frequently in males than females by a ratio of 2 to 1.

Astrocytomas arising from the cerebellum usually carry a better prognosis than those arising from the cerebrum. This is probably due to the fact that cerebellar astrocytomas give rise to symptons earlier. Furthermore these are predominantly of the piloid variety in which approximately 75 per cent tend to be cystic tumors relatively not invasive. In view of such characteristics, cerebellar astrocytomas often lend themselves to complete surgical eradication. The operative mortality is low, often nil. Recurrences are relatively infrequent.

Following surgical removal alone, long-term survivals of 5 years or longer may be expected in approximately 75 to 80 per cent of the patients. Actually, in a series of 41 patients with cerebellar astrocytomas, Levy and Elvidge[67] have reported that treatment consisted of surgical removal exclusively in 29 of the 34 who were followed up. Subsequently to surgical removal alone 22 of 29 or 76 per cent of the patients have survived over 5 years up to 14, and most of them were still living at the time of their report. Of the 22 survivors, 4 were patients in whom tumor extirpation was considered incomplete.

Surgical removal followed with irradiation was the treatment applied in 5 of the 34 cerebellar astrocytomas reported in Levy and Elvidge's series. Removal had been considered complete in 2 and incomplete in 3 patients. The 5 patients who received postoperative irradiation in their series are included in our total series of 14 patients so treated. Of these 14 patients irradiated postoperatively for cerebellar astrocytomas 12 are surviving at present time and the survival range varies from 5 to 22 years: 3 patients have survived over 20 years, 2 over 15 years, 5 over 10 years, and 2 over 5 years. At the time of postoperative irradiation 8 of our 12 survivors were under 15 years of age, 3 other patients were under 20 and the remaining survivor was 30 years old. All 12 survivors (86 per cent) are in excellent condition mentally, and only one is physically partially disabled on account of an unsteady gait.

It is difficult to elicit the value of postoperative irradiation in the treatment of cerebellar astrocytomas in consideration of the high rate of long survivals (76 per cent of 29 patients reported by Levy and Elvidge) and satisfactory recoveries following surgical removal alone. The same workers have reported 4 5-year survivors among 7 patients whose tumors were considered incompletely removed and yet were not subjected to any additional treatment. On that account, survivals over 5 years may not have too much significance in relation to the potential value of postoperative irradiation of cerebellar astrocytomas because of incomplete surgical removal.

Postoperative irradiation of cerebellar astrocytomas might be indicated in 15 to 20 per cent of all cases, particularly in the cases of solid tumors which may not be completely eradicated surgically. Considering the localized nature, the small volume and low depth of cerebellar astrocytomas, small fields 5 x 5 to 6 x 8 cm. in size are usually adequate. The portal arrangement consists of 2 lateral and 1 posterior occipital fields. Crossfiring with Cobalt[60] radiation beams, tumor doses of 4500 to 5000 rads are administered over periods of 40 to 45 days.

Expanding lesions in the posterior fossa should not be irradiated unless a histological diagnosis is available prior to irradiation. This is particularly important because tumors in that location are largely found in the young under 15 years of age, their nature is variable and the therapeutic management differs with the type of tumor. Once a diagnosis of cerebellar astrocytoma is made or suspected, surgical management is indicated primarily.

In conclusion, the treatment of choice for cerebellar astrocytomas seems to consist of surgical removal alone. It is not clear that postoperative radiation may have contributed significantly to increase the longevity of patients when it has been administered to tumors considered incompletely removed. Our long-term results reported above are most gratifying in every respect insofar as survival and recovery rates are considered but reveal no statistically significant advantage over surgical treatment alone.

Gliomas of the Optic Chiasm and Nerves

These are tumors which are rather uncommon, and are considered congenital in nature. Tumors involving the optic chiasm and nerves are found mostly in children, but may appear in adults. These tumors that are usually growing slowly may become very large and fill the third ventricle. Histologically, chiasmatic tumors belong to the astrocytoma group and ordinarily are well differentiated. Kahn, Bassett, Schneider and Crosby[51] have reported an incidence of 1 per cent in 1577 brain tumors.

Because of their anatomic location, gliomas of the optic chiasm and nerves are not easily accessible for surgery. Davis and Davis[27] have stated that surgical experience with the chiasmatic spongiblastomas is discouraging, inasmuch as these tumors frequently involve the mid-brain as well as the chiasm. Kahn *et al.* have expressed the opinion that such tumors could not possibly respond to surgery and, since they are astrocytic and spongioblastic growths, it does not seem reasonable to suppose that they would respond to x-ray therapy.

Poppen[90] believes that if only one side is involved the tumor should be removed, but only when the patient is blind in that eye. In the opinion of Poppen, x-ray therapy is of real help in some cases.

Dyke and Davidoff[26] reported 4 cases of glioma of the optic chiasm and nerves. Three were explored surgically so that the presence of tumors was verified, but biopsy was taken in just one of these and this proved to be an astrocytoma. They stated that all these cases have shown improvement, sometimes of remarkable degree and of long duration, and they concluded that this must be ascribed to radiation therapy beyond any doubt.

The results of MacCarty[72] in the treatment of 10 astrocytomas of the optic mechanism and hypothalamus present a markedly different experience from that just reported. All tumors in his series were low-grade astrocytomas except for one. At the time of his report, 9 patients were alive including 3 who had survived for 5 years and 1 for 7 years. Total removal was accomplished in 2, and one of these was irradiated prophylactically following surgery. In the 7 patients who had only a partial removal, some form of radiation therapy was administered.

Our own experience with gliomas arising from the optic chiasm and nerves is limited to 3 patients treated more than 5 years ago, 2 children and 1 adult. One of the children is alive and well 10 years following combined treatment by surgical removal and postoperative intensive irradiation. The other child was found to have a very large tumor at the base of the brain, obstructing the aqueduct. At operation, biopsy only could be taken and this revealed an astrocytoma. A shunt was established and a tumor dose of nearly 5000 rads was administered in 45 days. The child survived 27 months but was almost completely blind. At autopsy, an astrocytoma of the optic chiasm and nerves was found. The adult patient survived only 10 months after treatment. Not included in our present series is the recent case of a large chiasmatic glioma in a child who survived only 2 years after removal and irradiation.

Treatment planning must vary according to the size of the lesion insofar as the position and size of the fields are concerned, but we rely largely on opposing lateral fields. Tumor doses must be adequate but well protracted because of the vulnerabiity of adjacent hypothalamic and thalamic structures. High energy radiation should be used and tumor doses of not less than 6000 rads over 50 to 60 days should be administered.

The evidence reviewed above regarding the management and results in gliomas arising from the optic chiasm and optic nerves makes it clear that the prognosis is rather unpredictable. The opinions and results reported are at considerable variance. The degree of histologic differentiation, the rate of growth and the impact on adjacent structures must be responsible for such contrasting experiences. It would seem that thorough clinical investigation and surgical exploration are essential to ascertain the diagnosis and remove the tumor to an extent dictated by the experience and wisdom of the surgeon. Adequate intensive but protracted postoperative irradiation should be administered in all cases, as it might be beneficial and unlikely to induce adverse effects.

Overall Long-Term Survival Rates Following Adequate Irradiation of Intracranial Astrocytomas

In the total series of intracranial gliomata that we have treated and followed up for more than 5 years, astrocytomas account for exactly 123 cases or 25 per cent. Irradiation was used postoperatively in 120. Only 3 patients were treated with radiation alone. The majority of astrocytomas involved the cerebral hemispheres including 9 cases irradiated only at the time of recurrence following surgical treatment alone. The rest of the total group comprises 14 cerebellar and 3 optic nerves astrocytomas. There are no astrocytomas of the mid-brain or pons included in the total group. All cases were verified histologically.

The overall survival rates (Table 4) demonstrate that patients with astrocytomas have a better prognosis and higher life expectancy than the other intracranial gliomata of astrocytic origin irradiated in the course of their treatment.

GLIOMAS OF OLIGODENDROCYTIC ORIGIN

Oligodendrogliomas, tumors arising from the oligodenrogliocytes, are not frequent. Other equivalent terminology consists of the following: oligodendrocytoma, fusocellular oligodendrocytoma, gliome à petites cellules rondes, schwannoid oligodendrogliomas. These tumors are found mostly in the cerebellar hemispheres of young adults, occasionally in middle-aged people, rarely in children. Oligodendrogliomas have the lowest incidence of all primary intracranial gliomata. These tumors are known to be usually slow-growing, well circumscribed and relatively benign. Oligodendrogliomas often contain numerous deposits of calcium which can be identified frequently on plain x-ray films of the skull. Some of these tumors are classified as oligodendroglioblastomas because of their more malignant appearance since they grow faster and histologically exhibit larger round cells with occasional mitoses.

Reports on the treatment of relatively large groups of oligodendrogliomas are few. Horrax[45] has reported 31 cases in which the tumor was extirpated surgically and 11 of his patients had a useful survival for 5 to 31 years, a 34 per cent rate. From 18 patients available for follow-up MacCarty[72] reported a 5-year survival rate of 44 per cent following surgical removal.

Our series of cases irradiated postoperatively comprises only 14 patients. These received roentgen therapy following surgical removal either because of the more malignant histological appearance than usual or in view of surgical extirpation definitely incomplete. Actual survivals show that one half of the patients (7) irradiated, all postoperatively, have survived over 5 years. From these, 3 of 9 patients irradiated over 10 years ago are still living and 1 of them treated more than 20 years ago is alive and well. All patients surviving over 5 years have made a good recovery and remained well from the time of irradiation.

Considering that oligodendrogliocytic tumors usually are well differentiated and are probably not overly radiosensitive, they should be treated with megavoltage radiation and tumor doses of approximately 6500 rads in 50 to 60 days.

From our limited experience in dealing with oligodendrogliomas and oligodendroglioblastomas I find it difficult to determine to what extent postoperative irradiation may contribute to longer and better survivals in comparison with surgical removal alone. The number of cases is too small (only 9 patients irradiated more than 10 years ago) to allow for any comparison which might be truly significant and reveal more than a trend.

GLIOMAS OF EPENDYMAL CELL ORIGIN

Ependymomas and ependymoblastomas are tumors representing a group of neoplasms arising from the ependymal lining of the ventricular system. Neuropathologists are using a rich nomenclature to designate tumors in this histological category. Synonymous terminology may be as follows: ependymal glioma, glioependymoma, glioepithelioma, medulloepithelioma, neuroepithelioma, papilloma of the choroid plexus, and some neuroblastomas.

Tumors developing from ependymal cells and tissue may be found anywhere along the ventricular system. The majority of them grow slowly and are histologically benign. The minority, approximately 15 to 20 per cent, are classed as ependymoblastomas when histologically they show tumor cells of embryonal type with increased mitotic activity, and biologically they appear to grow faster than usual. Zimmerman et al.[123] consider that ependymal cell tumors are usually not completely removable and that recurrence is frequent even after surgical removal considered complete. French[37] is of the opinion that all ependymomas, except the papillomas, are fundamentally malignant because of their invasive tendencies. The incidence of intracranial ependymal tumors is low. Zulch[127] with his co-workers classified more than 6000 intracranial tumors and found 259 ependymomas, an incidence of 4.3 per cent. Ependymomas are seen mostly in children and young adults, and also in the fifth decade of life. The duration of symptoms prior to diagnosis and treatment varies with their location, as these tumors grow predominantly within the ventricular cavities that the tumor may fill.

The exact diagnosis of ependymal tumors cannot be made ordinarily without surgical exploration. At the same time, extirpation of as much tumor as feasible should constitute the initial treatment in all cases. Neurosurgeons generally agree that complete surgical removal of ependymomas and ependymoblastomas, whether supratentorial or infratentorial, cannot be accomplished safely in the majority of cases. This is due to their anatomical location and invasive tendency. Buchanan[16] and others have expressed the opinion that radiation has some effect on their growth and that life expectancy of children with ependymomas of the fourth ventricle is indefinite.

Dissemination Along Cerebrospinal Spaces

Ependymal cell tumors are reported to spread along the cerebrospinal spaces just like medulloblastomas do. On that basis, Dyke and Davidoff[26] have advocated prophylactic doses of radiation to the entire spinal axis in the treatment of histologically verified ependymomas, either of the cerebrum or the cerebellum. In previous articles([14])([15]) we have stated that in the management of ependymomas our practice has been not to irradiate routinely the spinal axis.

At present our series comprises 20 patients treated over 5 years ago for intracranial ependymal cell tumors. The primary location was supratentorial in 17, and infratentorial in the remaining 3 cases. From histological studies, 14 were classified in the ependymoma and 6 in the ependymoblastoma subgroups. Postoperative irradiation was concentrated at the site of the primary tumor. The spinal axis was irradiated prophylactically in the manner suggested by Dyke and Davidoff[26] in 2 cases only. Patients have been followed from 5 to more than 20 years from the onset of radiation therapy. Clinical evidence of neoplastic dissemination and implant along the spinal subarachnoid spaces has not been observed as yet in any of the 20 patients that we have irradiated postoperatively.

Kricheff, Becker, Schneck and Taveras[61] are also of the opinion that prophylactic irradiation of the spinal axis is not indicated following treatment of histologically verified intracranial ependymomas. From a series of 70 proven cases, 59 patients were available for follow-up exceeding 5 years. The location of tumors was supratentorial in 14 and infratentorial in 45 cases. Involvement of the spinal cord with metastases was suspected clinically in one case only, 6 years after initial treatment, but this was never verified as no autopsy was performed. This was 1 of the 4 patients whose spinal axis they had irradiated prophylactically after operation. Postmortem examination of spinal cords in 12 of their cases revealed no evidence of implants from the primary ependymomas.

Svien, Gates and Kernohan[110] have studied the spinal cords from 19 patients who had intracranial ependymomas. They found subarachnoid implants in 6 cases, but none of the patients had ever shown clinical evidence such that the presence of the neoplastic implants in the cord could be suspected. It is difficult to reconcile the contrasting difference between the autopsy findings of Svien et al.[110] and those reported by Kricheff and his associates[61]. The observations of Svien et al. suggest that the incidence of spinal cord implants may be higher than that of clinically detected cases, but this is not corroborated by the series of autopsies mentioned above (Kricheff et al.). Our series contains no autopsy material. It would seem, however, that disseminated and implanted ependymal cells had ample time to grow and manifest themselves clinically, considering that 20 patients in our series of ependymomas were treated over 5 years ago and some followed up to 10, 15, 20 years and longer (Table 4). We agree with Kricheff et al. that clinical evidence of spread of intracranial ependymomas along the spinal cord is quite rare. Accordingly, we also share their opinion that no need exists for prophylactic irradiation of the entire central nervous axis at the time of treatment of the primary tumor.

Treatment Results in Supratentorial and Infratentorial Ependymomas

Assessment of the most efficacious method for treating primary intracranial ependymomas and ependymoblastomas can be derived from the study of immediate and long-term results. Surgical treatment is essential primarily. It is needed first as the exact diagnosis is ordinarily made at the time of craniotomy. At the same time pressure phenomena associated with most ependymal cell tumors will be relieved. Surgical removal of tumor may be used alone and postoperative survivors may be subjected to adequate irradiation as an added therapeutic procedure. There seems to be virtually no place for treatment with radiation alone. Chemotherapeutic agents remain untried in this category of gliomas.

Results in 54 patients treated exclusively with surgical extirpation of intracranial ependymomas have been reported by Ringertz and Reymond[99]. From 21 patients operated for supratentorial ependymomas, 13 survived operation and were followed up adequately. Of these 13 patients, who each had the chance of surviving over 5 years, only 2 have actually

TABLE 7. Intracranial Ependymomas

Five-Year Survival Rates Related to Location of Tumor and
Treatment by Surgical Removal Alone or Postoperative Irradiation

Method of Treatment	Supratentorial			Infratentorial			All Ependymomas		
	No. of Patients	5 Year Survivors	Per cent	No. of Patients	5 Year Survivors	Per cent	No. of Patients	5 Year Survivors	Per cent
Surgical removal alone Ringertz and Reymond	13	2	15	15	5	35	28	7	25
Surgical removal and adequate irradiation									
(a) Kricheff, Becker, Schneck and Taveras	9	2	22	33	15	45	42	17	41
(b) Bouchard and Associates	17	11	65	3	3	100	20	14	70

exceeded that length of a time, a 5-year survival rate of 15 per cent (Table 7). Among 33 patients with infratentorial ependymomas, 30 were operated and 15 survived surgical intervention. Of these 15 postoperative survivors available for follow-up, 5 have lived over 5 years, a survival rate of 35 per cent.

In summarizing the surgical experience of Ringertz and Reymond, it appears that altogether 28 of 54 patients have survived operation and could have been exposed to postoperative irradiation, but none of them was. Of these 28 potential 5-year survivors treated with surgical removal exclusively, 7 have actually lived more than 5 years, giving a net 5-year survival rate of 25 per cent (Table 7). Local recurrences took place in 7 of the 13 patients who survived a first operation and had had an apparently complete removal of supratentorial ependymomas. In 6 of the 15 patients who survived incomplete extirpation of infratentorial tumors, local recurrence developed. The degree of clinical recovery is not indicated.

Review of 41 patients treated with surgical removal and postoperative irradiation for intracranial ependymomas and followed for 5 years or longer, from the time of diagnosis, has been reported by Kricheff and Associates[61]. Of 9 potential 5-year survivors so treated for supratentorial tumors, 2 patients have actually survived over 5 years, a rate of 22 per cent (Table 7). Among the 33 patients treated for infratentorial ependymomas who could have lived 5 years or longer, 15 actually did, a 5-year survival rate of 45 per cent. The overall 5-year survival rate is 41 per cent. The quality of survival, estimated 1 year from the time of diagnosis, is rated as excellent and good in 5 of 10 patients treated for supratentorial tumors and in 27 of 35 patients treated for infratentorial tumors. The rate of incidence of local recurrences among the 41 patients has not been brought out distinctly from the discussion on recurrences, but it would appear to be rather high.

Our own series comprises 20 patients who were treated by surgical operation followed by adequate irradiation for intracranial ependymomas and ependymoblastomas. All were followed for at least 5 years from the onset of postoperative irradiation. Among 17 patients treated for supratentorial tumors, 11 or 65 per cent have survived over 5 years (Table 7). The 3 patients treated for infratentorial tumors are still living 18, 19, and 22 years respectively after radiation therapy.

The overall 5-year survival rate in our cases is 70 per cent, since 14 of 20 patients have survived over 5 years from the onset of postoperative irradiation (Table 7). It should be added that 10 of 18 have survived over 10 years, 7 of 12 have exceeded 15 years of survival, and 3 of 7 are living over 20 years (Table 4). Of the patients now deceased, 2 have not improved following treatment and 6 died of local recurrences.

The quality of survival among our patients was good (Grade I recovery) for 5 years or longer in 11 of 14 survivors and remained such for those among the 11 who have survived over 10, 15 or 20 years. The other 3 patients were partially disabled at the time irradiation was commenced and remained so, 2 over 15 years and the other over 20 years. One of these 3 patients has recently become totally disabled from local recurrence.

Factors Influencing Prognosis

Supratentorial or Infratentorial Location:—The prognosis of patients with intracranial ependymomas appears to be influenced by certain factors. The intracranial location of a primary ependymal cell tumor, whether supratentorial or infratentorial, is recognized in most reports as an important element in relation to treatment results. From their experience, Kricheff and Associates[61] believe that patients with supratentorial ependymomas have the worse prognosis (Table 7) and have greater neurological deficits than patients with infratentorial tumors. Their opinion is partly corroborated by the results of Ringertz and Reymond[99] who, out of 13 patients, had only 2 survivors for 5 years or longer following treatment solely with surgical removal. These authors have also observed that ependymomas arising from the floor of the fourth ventricle usually carry a bad prognosis.

Our series is comprising supratentorial ependymomas predominantly (17 cases). These tumors were primarily hemispheral. Two ependymal cell tumors arising from the third ventricle are not included here, but are classed with mid-brain tumors. Otherwise, our series includes only 3 infratentorial ependymomas. The length of survival and degree of recovery have been excellent in all 3 patients treated for infratentorial ependymomas. This may be used in support of the opinion of Kricheff *et al.*[61] who believe that results of treatment are better in the infratentorial tumors from the time that patients can be considered as postoperative survivors.

Survival rates in the 3 comparative series of cases presented in Table 7 demonstrate clearly that the prognosis of patients who have survived operation is better among those who had infratentorial ependymomas in contrast with supratentorial tumors. It must be emphasized that operative and immediate postoperative mortality has been high. The survival rates presented in Table 7 do not reflect the morbidity of this particular category of gliomas. These rates merely represent an actual proportion of patients who, having survived operation, have lived 5 years or longer and could then become the subjects for a study of treatment results. Such study is available in Table 7, in relation to the anatomic location of intracranial ependymomas and in relation also to the method of treatment applied whether it be surgery alone or surgery combined with postoperative irradiation. This comparison must be valid, considering that those survival rates have emerged solely from patients who had survived surgical removal and the immediate postoperative period (approximately 1 month after operation). Those patients could then become available for follow-up, and were actually traced in their clinical path.

Histologic Factors—Ependymoblastomas. The influence of histologic variations on prognosis have been pointed out by Ringertz and Reymond.[99] They have stated that in malignant ependymomas or ependymoblastomas the prognosis seems to be more severe than in histologically benign ependymomas. Recurrences are seen earlier and more frequently in ependymoblastomas, resulting in lower survival and shorter periods of good recovery.

In our series of ependymal cell tumors, 6 were considered malignant and classed as ependymoblastomas, all arising from the supratentorial region. Of these 6 patients, one did not respond to radiation therapy and died within 5 months, whereas another who improved clinically died from recurrence less than 2 years after initiation of postoperative radiation therapy. Three of the 6 patients barely survived 5 years, and each of them had to be treated for recurrence once or twice in the course of their respective survival periods. Such survival periods were relatively short in comparison with those observed in patients treated for less malignant ependymal cell tumors. The remaining patient survived 9 years without local recurrence and in good clinical condition before dying of bronchopneumonia.

Influence of Age Factor. In the opinion of Kricheff *et al.,*[61] prognosis is worse in children than in adults affected with intracranial ependymomas. In their total series of 69 children, 25 per cent have survived longer than 3 years, in contrast with 45 per cent of 33 adults who have survived 3 years also. Our experience differs from that of Kricheff *et al.*[61] but is less significant, considering that ours is based upon results observed in a much smaller group of children.

From our series of 20 ependymomas, 7 occurred in children and all were supratentorial. Of these 7 children, 5 survived over 3 years. In the adult group, 7 of 10 patients with supratentorial ependymal cell tumors were living at the end of the 3-year period. Comparison of the 3-year survival rates between children and adults treated for supratentorial ependymal cell tumors reveals no significant difference. Four of the children irradiated postoperatively have now reached adulthood and are alive and well: 2 over 10 years, 1 over 15 and the other over 20 years. It may be interesting to add that 3 of the 6 cases of supratentorial ependymoblastomas were in children. They had relatively short survivals as they lived respectively 5, 22 and 62 months following treatment.

Technique of Irradiation

Ependymomas and ependymoblastomas have been treated in our series with kilovoltage X-radiation. We have been using a crossfiring arrangement consisting of anterior and lateral pairs of opposing fields. In a single course of daily treatments, 5 days a week, tumor doses of 5000 rads delivered over 45 to 50 days have been administered. The younger children have received tumor doses of 4500 to 5000 rads and the older were given depth doses equal to those administered to adults over the same average period of time. With megavoltage, total tumor doses should be increased by 500 to 1000 rads over the same period of time for treatment.

Kricheff et al.[61] have been using repeated courses of treatment but have changed over to a single protracted course of kilovoltage roentgen therapy over the last decade. Their plan of treatment is now consisting of tumor doses of 4000 rads in 4 weeks or 5000 rads in 6 weeks. In treating children, they use a modification of Richmond's schedule of doses such that infants receive 50 per cent of the dose given to adults, the 5-year old children are exposed to 75 per cent of the dose, whereas those exceeding 8 years of age are treated with the full dose. Kricheff et al.[61] report that 20 autopsies were performed in patients with ependymomas, supratentorial in 6 cases, at different times following radiation therapy. No evidence of radiation necrosis outside of the tumor could be related to tumor doses varying from 2000 to 4000 rads in 3 to 4 weeks.

Recurrence of Intracranial Ependymal Cell Tumors

Local intracranial recurrence of ependymomas and ependymoblastomas is the usual cause of death in patients who have survived a first operation in the treatment of their primary condition. Pool, Ransohoff and Correll[89] believe that multiple operations over long periods of time may be successful, with or without radiation therapy. Kricheff et al.[61] have treated local recurrences of ependymomas with additional irradiation. It is their opinion that the danger inherent to regrowth of tumor is far greater than that of damage to normal brain from repeated radiation treatments. In the management of ependymomas which have recurred and had been irradiated previously, following surgical removal, they advocate smaller doses in the range of 1800 to 2000 rads in 2 to 3 weeks. They have re-treated more than once as the need arose.

In our series, 4 patients were treated for recurrent ependymal cell tumors. Re-irradiation was accomplished with tumor doses of 3000 rads over 6 weeks in 2 patients, and 6000 rads in 7 to 8 weeks in a third patient. In the first 2 patients, signs of clinical improvement and tumor regression were observed for periods of time varying from 1 to 2 years. No improvement occurred in the third case. The most recent recurrence was an ependymoblastoma which was not re-irradiated but re-operated. This patient recovered nicely for a period extending practically over 2 years, and then another recurrence developed which was treated by a third surgical removal but the subsequent remission was of shorter duration and she died less than 2 years later from further recurrence.

Clinical surgical staging of infratentorial ependymomas is advocated by

Kricheff and associates. They believe this can be done at the time of operation and determined from the extent of the tumor together with the degree of invasion of the surrounding brain. This may be of prognostic value in their opinion.

In summary, from the evidence accumulated regarding the management of primary intracranial ependymomas and ependymoblastomas, the following conclusions seem to emerge.

Surgical removal and subsequent adequate radiation therapy afford patients a greater chance of good recovery with longer survival than surgical extirpation alone. Surgical removal is rarely complete and is often followed by local recurrences. Radiation therapy should be directed to the primary tumor site. There is definitely no need for prophylactic irradiation of the spinal axis for the control of potential tumor spread and implants which rarely manifest themselves clinically. Local recurrences may be re-treated by irradiation or subjected to a second surgical removal, and good remission can be obtained from either method.

Prognosis is more favorable in the infratentorial and also the histologically low malignancy ependymomas, but perhaps not as good in children as in adults. High survival and good recovery rates may be anticipated as results of adequate control of primary growth. Treatment of recurrences may bring further periods of remission and useful survival. We agree with Kricheff and associates that the effects of radiation therapy are variable in ependymal cell tumors, and that it is impossible to predict which tumor classed in the ependymal cell category of gliomas may or may not respond to radiation.

On the basis of long-term treatment results, we believe that all ependymomas and ependymoblastomas should be irradiated postoperatively.

MEDULLOBLASTOMA

Of all primary intracranial tumors, medulloblastomas are recognized as the most common type in children and also the most sensitive to ionizing radiation. Medulloblastoma is a widely accepted term in the nomenclature of tumors of the central nervous system, but the following terms are considered synonymous: neuroblastoma, glioblastoma isomorphe, and neurogliocytome embryonnaire.

There is no agreement amongst neuropathologists regarding the histogenesis of medulloblastomas. These usually arise in the posterior fossa of the cranial cavity, mostly from the mid-line of the cerebellum. Some neuropathologists believe that medulloblastoma is a tumor of glial origin, and this concept appears to rally the majority of opinions. Others believe that medulloblastomas arise from neuroblasts. Elvidge, Penfield and

Cone[31] have expressed the opinion that "both neuronal and neuroglial elements can be traced with fair certainty within some of these tumors and that many cells appear at a somewhat younger stage of development. This would seem to justify the term medulloblast, signifying that differentiation might proceed along either of the two lines". Electron microscopists might soon solve this dilemma but have not as yet, to my knowledge. Recently Luse[71], having studied 5 medulloblastomas by electron microscopy, stated that the exact cell of origin of this enigmatic tumor is not known.

Histopathologic Differential Diagnosis

Microscopically, medulloblastomas often are difficult to differentiate from cerebellar sarcomas and at times from ependymoblastomas. Smith, Lampe, and Kahn[106] have presented 4 eminent neuropathologists with histologic sections of tumors identified as medulloblastomas. The tumor sections provided for opinion originated from 5 cases in which postoperative results were exceptionally good. Two of the 4 pathologists declared that all tumors are medulloblastomas. A third pathologist believed that sections 1 to 4 are all medulloblastomas but section 5 is not. A fourth pathologist thought that section 1 was typical medulloblastoma with standard stain but more suggestive of an alveolar sarcoma in Perdrau stain for reticulin; section 2 was probably representing an alveolar sarcoma; sections 3 and 4 showed definite alveolar sarcomas; he interpreted section 5 as a neuro-spongioblastoma. This clearly illustrates how difficult it is among expert neuropathologists to classify tumors into separate histologic categories, when microscopically they may resemble one another so closely.

From the clinical standpoint, cerebellar or alveolar sarcomas cannot be distinguished from medulloblastomas in children, in the opinion of Smith, Lampe and Kahn[106]. On histopathologic examination the distinction is usually made on the basis of reticulin stain, and obviously this is a controversial subject. They suggest in their article that "it should seem preferable to class them altogether as medulloblastomas of different unpredictable degrees of malignancy rather than to change the diagnosis the day the patient survives 5 years".

Incidence and Morbidity

The incidence of medulloblastomas in relation to all intracranial tumors was 3.8 per cent in the 6000 cases classified by Zulch[127] and his co-workers. Berger and Elvidge[10] have reported an incidence of 4.05 per cent or 109 cases from 2443 intracranial tumors diagnosed and treated at the Montreal Neurological Institute over a 30-year period, 1928 to 1958. When incidence is estimated in relation to intracranial gliomata only, the incidence reported is 6.7 per cent of 1522 cases. Cerebellar astrocytomas showed an incidence of 5.46 per cent. In our series of 494 irradiated primary intracranial gliomata, medulloblastomas account for 10 per cent of the cases.

The medulloblastoma is a neoplastic entity which was first identified and described in 1925 by Bailey and Cushing[6]. These outstanding neuro-surgeons were not long to recognize that this tumor is very anaplastic and highly malignant in behavior. The outcome of untreated medulloblastoma is rapidly fatal. They also realized that the most radical surgical extirpation is seldom complete and usually incapable of modifying a hopeless prognosis. Bailey and Cushing soon became aware that medulloblasts are most vulnerable to irradiation and that radiation therapy is definitely beneficial in prolonging the average postoperative survival.

Medulloblastomas are known to have a natural tendency to spread within the subarachnoid and ventricular spaces. This was first noted by Bailey and Cushing[6] who found metastases attached to the meninges along the spinal canal and advocated systematic irradiation of the spinal axis in all cases. This practice is well established and remains valid.

REVIEW OF TREATMENT METHODS

Surgical Extirpation Alone

In 1936, Cutler, Sosman and Vaughan[24] compiled the results of treatment in 61 cases of medulloblastomas that Cushing had reported in 1930. Deaths were recorded in 21 patients, 2 untreated and 19 who had died from operation. Among those who survived operation and could be followed, 14 patients subjected to no other treatment but surgical removal gave an average postoperative duration of life of 5.6 months. This was in contrast with an average of 6.7 months in 12 cases treated by irradiation postoperatively even though the radiation therapy administered was considered inadequate by Cutler *et al*. Three patients were found to have survived an average of 34.8 months subsequent to irradiation of the spinal axis and ventricular system in addition to their operation.

Many surgeons have reported discouraging results in the management of cerebellar medulloblastomas with surgery alone. Berger and Elvidge[10] have reported an average survival barely exceeding 1 year in 14 patients operated upon who had no radiotherapy postoperatively. Recently, Smith, Lampe, and Kahn have stated in relation to medulloblastomas that "the futility of attempting cure by radical operation has become established".

Surgical Removal Followed by Irradiation

The high operative mortality rate and the inefficacy of surgical procedures alone in the control of cerebellar medulloblastomas have been generally recognized. The effectiveness of X-radiation as a complement to operative procedures in the treatment of primary medulloblastoma, its recurrences or metastases, was acknowledged by Cushing himself.

Irradiation, however, should not be administered upon a presumptive diagnosis of medulloblastoma. Histopathologic proof is essential to guide the surgeon in determining the procedure to follow and the radiotherapist in selecting the appropriate method of irradiation.

It is generally considered that radiation therapy should follow an operation at which histological verification is obtained and decompression accomplished by removal of tumor tissue. The degree of tumor extirpation may vary with the extent of the growth and the wisdom of the neurosurgeon. The fear that surgical procedures may be responsible for the dissemination of tumor cells along the subarachnoid spaces should not be slighted because such spread can occur without surgery, according to reports by Abbott and Kernohan[1] and also by Cairns and Russell.[17]

Paterson and Farr[82] have reported a 3-year survival rate of 65 per cent in a series of 27 patients operated upon and irradiated for medulloblastomas between 1941 and 1950, and a 5-year survival of 30 per cent in 6 children among the 21 in that group who had been treated for more than 5 years. Richmond[97] reported his experience with the treatment of 110 children. Subtentorial gliomata predominated. Statistical analysis of his material has shown a 43 per cent 5-year survival in medulloblastomas.

Smith, Lampe and Kahn[106] have reported 61 cases of cerebellar medulloblastomas ranging in age from 9 weeks to 15 years, with the usual predominance of males over females. The operative and postoperative mortality was 20 per cent or 11 of the 56 patients who were operated initially. Altogether 41 children received postoperative irradiation under their supervision. Of these 41 patients, 38 were treated 5 or more years prior to their report and 11 or 28 per cent have survived for periods ranging from 5 to 17 years without known recurrence. Six of the 11 patients have survived over 10 years and this represents 21 per cent of those irradiated 10 years or longer before their report. From the standpoint of clinical recovery, out of the 38 children irradiated more than 5 years before review, 5 or 13 per cent were essentially normal.

In the opinion of Smith et al., repeated courses of postoperative irradiation did not seem greatly beneficial in general. They have changed their technique since 1950 because of a high incidence of mental retardation and seizures. Since then, they treated children with more protracted and fractionated irradiation of the entire ventricular system including the primary site, supplemented with moderate doses through the spinal canal concurrently. Of 8 children so treated, 5 were still living at the time of their report (1961), more than 5 years after onset of treatment. Except for the presence of metastases, no factor has been found to be of particular value in predicting the clinical course in a given case. In the treatment of

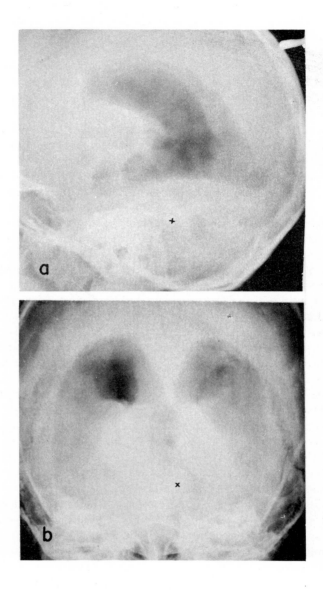

Figure 6 a, On ventriculograms, there is dilatation of third and lateral ventricles. (a) Lateral view shows an opaque round shadow (x) partly outlined with a thin rim of gas. This shadow was due to a tumor occupying most of the 4th ventricle leaving only the posterior and left portions opened.

b, On postero-anterior view the same space-occupying lesion as seen on (a) and marked with (x) is visualized in the fourth ventricle leaving just a faint outline of gas in the left part of the cavity.

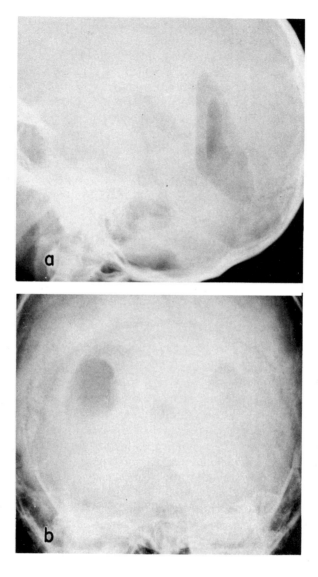

Figure 7 a, b, Same cases as 6 a and b.—Posterior fossa pneumoencephalograms made immediately after radiation therapy was completed demonstrate clear outline with gas of cisterna magna, fourth ventricle, aqueduct and most of the third ventricle, indicating free communication between spinal canal and ventricular system. The tumor mass has dissappeared.

Aspiration biopsy had revealed cerebellar medulloblastoma in a 7½ year old child. Following adequate irradiation of intracranial (4800 r/30 days) and spinal canal contents (1800 r/14 days) symptoms and signs disappeared. Patient presently alive and well, with family of four, 19 years after treatment.

cerebellar medulloblastomas, Smith, Lampe and Kahn[106] are now advocating operation followed by irradiation through the entire cerebrospinal axis in a single protracted course.

Results of treatment of cerebellar medulloblastomas are no longer hopeless as they used to be, a change which may be attributed to radiation therapy. Such improvement is not attributable, however, to the advent of high energy sources of ionizing radiation or megavoltage, since most reports indicate that patients with medulloblastomas have been treated with kilovoltage X-radiation. Better treatment planning and more adequate irradiation in relation to the time-dose-volume factors would appear to be the predominant elements which may have influenced better results among patients exposed to radiation therapy postoperatively. Using the technical advantages of megavoltage for adequate irradiation might contribute to further rise in better treatment results.

Treatment by Irradiation Alone

Radiation therapy is the only therapeutic agent which at present appears to be capable of curing medulloblastomas, therefore the only hope. The potential curative role of X-radiation used alone has been visualized for some time and prompted several workers to try and dispense with ineffective surgical removal and operative mortality.

Cutler, Sosman and Vaughan[24] reviewed a total of 81 cases of cerebellar medulloblastomas (including 61 cases of Cushing's series) and reported only 3 5-year survivors of whom only 1 was apparently free of disease at the time. They suggested to try and treat medulloblastomas by irradiation alone, avoiding even an exploratory operation and biopsy. Irradiation alone could be used in certain selected cases as a therapeutic test for differentiating medulloblastomas from other tumors of the posterior fossa. If the response to radiation were rapid and the symptoms regressed promptly, they considered that this was indicative of medulloblastoma and the patient should be continued on irradiation alone. If it were the contrary, surgical exploration and histologic verification should be done. The proposal of Cutler et al. to treat cerebellar medulloblastomas without histologic verification, solely on the basis of a clinical diagnosis, was frowned upon and condemned by the majority of neurosurgeons and radiotherapists.

Treatment of cerebellar medulloblastomas by irradiation alone, without operation, but following aspiration biopsy and histologic proof of diagnosis was proposed by Peirce, Cone, Bouchard and Lewis[84]. The authors could not agree with Cutler et al. who had suggested that suspected cerebellar tumors be treated with radiation only without histologic diagnosis. It was considered that children would do as well, and perhaps better, if the trauma associated with surgical intervention could be avoided and operative mortality eliminated. Medulloblastomas could be identified histologically from other lesions arising in the posterior fossa and thus permit immediate initiation of roentgen therapy. Tumor tissue was obtained under local anesthesia through a twist drill hole by using a brain biopsy needle.

Our[84] preliminary results following irradiation alone were reported for the initial group of 5 children so treated after making the diagnosis of medulloblastoma through that method of brain biopsy. Clinical response and improvement was dramatic within 72 hours in 3 of the children and within 2 weeks in the other 2. Tumor regression was also demonstrated by pneumoencephalographic studies made upon completion of roentgen therapy (Fig. 6a, b and 7a, b). Long-term results of treatment by irradiation alone (Table 8) will be presented and discussed in a subsequent paragraph in relation to a total of 10 children treated not less than 5 years ago after histological verification of cerebellar medulloblastomas.

ANALYSIS OF OUR TREATMENT RESULTS IN
MEDULLOBLASTOMA

Our series of cerebellar medulloblastomas comprises 50 patients irradiated more than 5 years ago: 37 children aged 15 or less, and 13 patients over 15 years of age. Recently Smith, Lampe and Kahn[106] recalled that Bailey has expressed the opinion that cerebellar medulloblastomas occurred only in children under 15 years of age and have often been confused with leptomeningeal sarcomas found in adults. Whether or not medulloblastomas represent a neoplastic process following such rigid age demarcation may be a debatable point. However, in presenting our results for the period 1939 to 1958, it is intended to follow the suggestion of Smith *et al.* and, at this point, consider children separately from the overall group of cerebellar medulloblastomas.

Medulloblastomas in Children

In our series of 37 children with histologically proven cerebellar medulloblastoma (Table 8), treatment in 27 cases has consisted of surgical removal, more of less radical, followed by irradiation of the entire intracranial and spinal canal content. Irradiation alone was used in 10 children who, prior to initiation of radiation therapy, had had an aspiration biopsy for histological verification of their tumor.

Results in children are shown (Table 8) by the proportion of survivors after 1, 3, 5, 10, 15 and 20 years in relation to the method of treatment, either by surgery plus irradiation or by irradiation alone.

In children irradiated postoperatively, our survival rates are 33 per cent over 3 years, 22 per cent over 5 years, and 13 per cent over 10 years.

TABLE 8.   Cerebellar Medulloblastomas in Children*
Results by Method of Treatment and Survival

| Method of Treatment | 1 Year | *Proportion of Survivors Over* | | | | |
		3 Years	5 Years	10 Years	15 Years	20 Years
Surgical Removal and Irradiation	17/27	9/27	6/27	3/23	1/17	0/5
Needle Biopsy and Irradiation Only	8/10	4/10	4/10	2/7	1/4	0/1
Overall Survivals	25/37	13/37	10/37	5/30	2/21	0/6
Average Rates	70%	35%	27%	17%	10%	0%

* All patients of 15 years of age or under—every case verified histologically. At the end of each 5-year period, Grade I recovery for all survivors except one partially disabled at 5 years.

Among the 27 children irradiated postoperatively, 5 had to be treated again because of tumor manifestations along the spinal cord. Perhaps irradiation had not been adequate along the spinal axis. Our results are neither as good as those reported by Paterson and Farr nor by Smith, Lampe and Kahn.

The number of children treated by irradiation alone for cerebellar medulloblastomas is relatively small (Table 8), but the proportion of long-term survivors among these is twice as high as it is among children irradiated postoperatively. As yet, not one of the 10 children who had radiation therapy alone more than 5 years ago has developed clinical evidence of seeding and implant of tumor cells along the subarachnoid cerebrospinal spaces.

In children, irrelevant of the method of irradiation, whether postoperative or alone, our overall long-term survival rates (Table 8) are as follow: 27 per cent over 5 years, 17 per cent over 10 years, and 10 per cent over 15 years. Of 6 potentiaal 20-year survivors, none has survived that long.

The degree of clinical recovery is such that 9 out of the 10 children, followed more than 5 years from the onset of irradiation, have grown and were living normally at the 5-year period of follow-up. One was partially disabled and died over 5 years from cardiac disease without evidence of recurrence of her medulloblastoma. The quality of survival of those living at 10 and 15 years after treatment has remained excellent all along, without recurrence.

Medulloblastoma in Adults

We have treated 13 patients exceeding age 15 for posterior fossa tumors diagnosed medulloblastomas. The age distribution was as follows at the time of treatment: 4 over 15 but under 20, 5 between 20 and 30, and 4 over 30.

In that group, treatment consisted of surgical removal plus postoperative irradiation in every case. Each patient was followed for at least 5 years from the onset of radiation therapy. Treatment results estimated by survival rates are practically identical to those obtained in children. Three of the 13 patients have survived over 5 years, 2 having died 7 and 10 years respectively after treatment, whereas the other is still living and working 22 years following postoperative irradiation. The 2 who died had made a good recovery and remained well for the major part of their survival.

We have participated in the treatment of 2 adults who have enjoyed exceptionally long survivals for 17 and 24 years respectively. The first case was reported by Penfield and Feindel[86] and the second has been mentioned by Berger and Elvidge[10]. In both cases, the diagnosis of medulloblastoma was made at the Montreal Neurological Institute where they were treated initially by surgical removal and subsequent postoperative irradiation. This was in 1928 and 1932 when the patients were 22 and 18 years of age respectively. These 2 adult patients were first treated many years before the beginning of the period under review but were irradiated for intracranial recurrence, under our supervision, in the late stages of their survival. Therefore they appear in our series of 13 adults treated for medulloblastomas only inasmuch as we have given them palliative irradiation after which they survived 15 and 51 months. For obvious reasons we could not include them among our long-term survivors.

Overall Results in Children and Adults

Our overall results indicate that the life expectancy of children and adults with cerebellar medulloblastoma (Table 9) is greater than it was in the past, when the average duration of life was approximately 6 months after surgery alone. Life expectancy is based upon the actual survivals of 50 patients (37 children and 13 adults) considered adequately irradiated for cerebellar medulloblastoma either postoperatively (40 cases) or solely

TABLE 9.   Cerebellar Medulloblastomas and Sarcomas
Comparison of Survival Rates Combined and Separately in Children or Adults

	No. of Cases	1 Year	3 Years	5 Years	10 Years	15 Years	20 Years
				Survival Rates Over			
Medulloblastomas—							
All Patients	50	74%	36%	27%	17%	9%	8%
Cerebellar Sarcomas—							
All Patients	12	83	75	58	30	66	0
Medullos and							
Sarcomas Combined	62	76	44	32	20	14	7
(a) in Children							
Only	42	70	40	30	18	14	0
(b) in Adults Only	20	90	50	40	24	15	15

All tumors were verified histologically—Treatment by irradiation alone in 10 medulloblastomas and 2 sarcomas. Surgical removal plus irradiation in 40 medulloblastomas and 10 sarcomas.

(10 cases). Every patient was followed for 5 years or longer up to 1964. A careful analysis of our results has demonstrated that survival rates are practically identical in either children or adults when overall children rates are considered separately (Table 8) in relation to the rates for all patients (Table 9).

Recovery was good for the greater part of the duration of survival among patients who lived less than 5 years after treatment. Recovery rates over 5 years have been most gratifying since only one of the long-term survivors was partially disabled.

Survival Rates in Children and Adults When Cerebellar Medulloblastomas and Sarcomas Are Considered in a Single Group

It was mentioned above that Smith, Lampe and Kahn believed that cerebellar sarcomas cannot be distinguished from medulloblastomas in children. In their opinion it should seem preferable to class them altogether as medulloblastomas of different unpredictable degrees of malignancy. We have attempted to determine and visualize to what degree our survival rates in medulloblastomas might be modified if we group them all together (Table 9) on the assumption that cerebellar sarcomas belong to the same histological class as medulloblastomas.

The survival rates from our 12 cerebellar sarcomas (5 in children and 7 in adults) are definitely higher than those from all medulloblastomas, although the number of sarcomas is relatively small for comparison purposes. Obviously (Table 9) the effect of merging all cerebellar sarcomas with all medulloblastomas would seem to result in better overall survival rates. The agglomeration of cerebellar medulloblastomas and sarcomas in patients of pediatric age, 15 or under, would give slightly higher survival rates than medulloblastomas alone in children (Table 8) but the difference would not be statistically significant. In the adult group the pooling of all medulloblastomas (13 cases) and cerebellar sarcomas (7 cases) would give survival rates significantly higher than the similar combination in children (Table 9).

If it should be agreed that, in children, cerebellar sarcomas may not be different from medulloblastomas and shall be classed together in the same histopathological group, then the entire cranial and spinal canal content should logically be irradiated. Perhaps such irradiation should also be done routinely by those who in children may continue to consider and classify cerebellar sarcomas independently from medulloblastomas. This technical approach would be indicated on account of the natural tendency that cerebellar sarcomas have to metastasize along the cerebrospinal fluid pathways, a characteristic observed by many and considered to be one that cerebellar sarcomas have in common with medulloblastomas.

The cranial and spinal canal content was irradiated in 3 of 4 patients now classed in the cerebellar sarcoma group. In these cases such irradiation happened by chance and not by design, since these children were originally diagnosed as medulloblastomas and treated as such before revision of diagnosis. Medulloblastomas are known not to metastasize outside of the central nervous system. Cerebellar sarcomas, in contrast, are recognized by Zimmerman[123] and others as having the ability to metastasize extracranially to bones, lungs, lymph nodes and other anatomic sites. It was primarily because of extracranial metastases proven at autopsy that the original diagnosis of medulloblastoma was revised to that of cerebellar sarcoma in the 3 cases that we have just mentioned.

Berger and Elvidge have reviewed 109 medulloblastomas and 20 cerebellar sarcomas which were treated at the Montreal Neurological Institute from 1928 to the end of 1958, over a period of 30 years. The majority of our cases happened to be incorporated in their study. The authors have come to the conclusion that the average survival time is longer in the sarcoma as compared with the medulloblastoma group. In their opinion, that difference is not statistically significant and can be explained by chance alone. Theirs is a good study for evaluation of the morbidity of medulloblastomas and cerebellar sarcomas side by side. There appears to be a substantial difference in the degree of morbidity of the two (Table 9).

From the initial 109 patients with cerebellar medulloblastomas, 12 or 11 per cent had survived over 5 years at the time of their report. Otherwise, 7 of 20 patients or 35 per cent had survived with cerebellar sarcomas over 5 years, and some of the patients had not been followed for 5 years as yet. They reported an operative mortality of 22 per cent in medulloblastomas.

Regarding the practice of twist drill biopsy, with or without radiotherapy, Berger and Elvidge have pointed out that it is not such an innocuous procedure as some may think, since death has occurred following that procedure in 3 patients with medulloblastomas.

RADIATION THERAPY TECHNIQUE

The technique of irradiation is of considerable importance in medulloblastomas. Irradiation to be adequate must include the entire intracranial content and not only the posterior fossa. It must at the same time include the entire content of the spinal canal. Megavoltage radiation from Cobalt[60] teletherapy units is currently used by us. Treatment should be delivered in a single course of protracted doses, over a total period of 45 to 50 days. During that period of time the entire intracranial content is exposed to a tumor dose of 5000 rads. The content of the entire spinal canal is irradiated concomitantly to the cranial cavity up to a tumor dose of 2000 rads during the initial 2 to 3 weeks of radiation therapy.

A modification of the technique used by Paterson and Farr[82] has been devised, by which the full cranial and spinal content is irradiated at once, in one stretch, through a single and properly shaped field (Plate 3, a and b). The patient is lying in prone position below a lead shielded screen resting on top of the treatment couch. A window, measuring 9 x 9 cm., has been cut over the posterior part of the head. In order to limit radiation exposure to the spinal cord and subarachnoid spaces, the opening in the shield narrows to a width of 4 cm. below the occiput and extends in the caudal direction to the level of the first sacral vertebra. Lead bricks are used to maintain the exposed field to the desired width. A multicurie Cobalt[60] source exposes the entire craniospinal area at a focus-skin distance of 125 cm. Adequate homogeneous exposure of the intracranial content to the desired tumor dose level is completed by adding an anterior field as shown on Plate 3, b. This is introduced as a separate field starting from the time that the spinal canal content has received the full tumor dose contemplated at that level.

We also use at times a moving field technique (Plate 3, c) in which both the table and the patient move longitudinally in relation to a perpendicular Cobalt[60] radiation beam which is stationary at a 50 cm. focus-skin distance. The other technical factors are identical to those described with the previous technique for adequate radiation exposure of the content of the skull and entire spinal canal.

Judicious utilization of cytotoxic or radiomimetic agents, such as cyclophosphamide, at the onset or over the full period of irradiation, would very likely enhance the direct radiation effect on cerebellar medulloblastomas. Initially, intravenous injections of substantial doses might be the most effective method. Oral administration daily and concurrently with radiation therapy would have the advantage of providing a more continuous combination of treatment for inhibiting tumor cell mitosis. It is our belief that systemic administration should be superior to intrathecal instillation in consideration of the probable inconsistency of distribution and concentration of the drug in the cerebrospinal fluid with the latter method. Knowing the well-established therapeutic value of ionizing radiation, it might be reasonably easy to assess over the years the usefulness of added chemotherapy in the management of cerebellar medulloblastomas. It is highly probable that this approach might contribute to higher recovery rates and longer survivals.

In conclusion, adequate irradiation at once of the entire content of the skull and spinal canal is essential in the treatment of cerebellar medulloblastoma. Surgical treatment alone is futile and completely unjustifiable. The great majority of neurosurgeons and therapeutic radiologists consider that radiation therapy should be used postoperatively. Irradiation must be adequate and administered in a single protracted course. The entire cranial and spinal content must be irradiated homogeneously, preferably through a single appropriately designed field.

PLATE 3

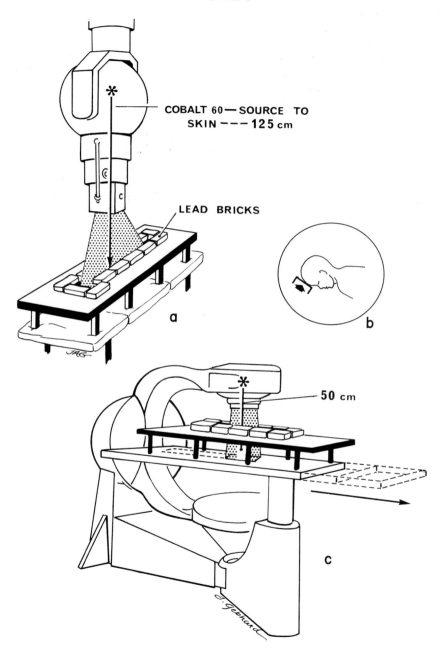

COBALT 60 — SOURCE TO
SKIN --- 125 cm

LEAD BRICKS

a

b

50 cm

c

Medulloblastoma—Irradiation of Entire Cerebrospinal Axis

117

Evidence has been presented that irradiation alone may be used success-fully without operation. Histological verification must be obtained prior to irradiation, and this can be procured by aspiration biopsy.

The encouraging results reported above in the management of medullo-blastomas are not based solely upon the dramatic clinical improvement that so many have witnessed in patients soon after the onset of radio-therapy. Long-term recovery and survival observations, recorded on pa-tients adequately treated with ionizing radiation postoperatively or alone, have brought accurate statistical studies to support a more optimistic trend. With adequate irradiation, good lasting recovery and long survivals may be expected for not less than 25 to 30 per cent of the children and adults treated for cerebellar medulloblastomas. The systematic utilization of cytotoxic or radiomimetic agents in combination with adequate radiation therapy might contribute to further improvement of long-term results.

6 Results of Radiation Therapy in Mid-Brain and Brain Stem Tumors

WHEN INTRACRANIAL TUMORS develop in the mid-brain or in the brain stem regions, the prognosis is considered unfavorable because of their anatomic location. Mid-brain tumors consist of neoplastic lesions arising in the anatomic region extending from the posterior portion of the third ventricle down to the pontine protuberance. The mid-brain is the crossroad of nearly all important motor and sensory nerve fibers where they converge on their way through the pons to the medulla. It also contains the aqueduct of Sylvius which controls the circulation of the cerebrospinal fluid within the brain itself. Nerve pathways emerge from the mid-brain into the brain stem or pons through which they establish a close anatomic liaison between the cerebrum, cerebellum and upper part of the medulla. There is no true anatomic division between the mid-brain and the pons, or between the pons and the upper part of the medulla. (Plate 4).

Incidence and Morbidity

Tumors growing in the mid-brain and pontine regions represent 14 per cent of all primary intracranial gliomata in our series of 494 primary intracranial gliomas. These tumors are infrequently accessible for biopsy. Ordinarily they cannot be extirpated surgically when explored, except at the cost of a high operative mortality. Unless the tumor should happen to be a glioblastoma multiforme, the important prognostic element is more the anatomic location of tumor growth than its histopathologic type. Untreated mid-brain and pontine tumors are predominantly fatal. Prolongation of life may be gained for a few patients with mid-brain tumors by relieving with shunts a dangerously increased intracranial pressure.

Histologic Diagnosis Dilemma

When clinical evidence indicates the presence of an expanding lesion located in the mid-brain or in the brain stem, the exact diagnosis may be accomplished by surgical exploration to try and obtain a biopsy. At the same time, treatment might be initiated if surgical removal can be attempted. If tumor extirpation cannot be performed, an aspiration biopsy may occasionally provide tissue diagnosis. The failure to obtain a definite histologic diagnosis by such surgical procedures often creates a dilemma. A decision has to be reached, to treat by irradiation alone without knowing the exact histologic nature of the suspected tumor, or not to treat on clinical evidence only. Gradually, through the years, a policy of compromise has been adopted.

There is considerable surgical and necropsy evidence that tumors growing in the mid-brain and pons are nearly always gliomata. We accept patients with mid-brain and brain stem tumors for treatment by irradiation alone, without the benefit of histologic confirmation and tumor classification, rather than risking a fatality. Otherwise histologic verification might become available only later, should there be a post-mortem examination. However, patients are accepted under such conditions only when a firm clinical diagnosis and a definite localization of the lesion are available.

The use of shunts to restore intraventricular circulation of cerebrospinal fluid and thus relieve increased intracranial pressure has contributed to reduce the incidence of complications. This is applicable particularly in the management of mid-brain tumors, perhaps not so much in pontine tumors. Our results suggest that adequate radiation therapy alone is capable of improving markedly the prognosis of mid-brain and pontine neoplasms.

Clinical Material

Our series comprises 37 mid-brain and 34 brain stem or pontine tumors, mostly treated by irradiation alone. Surgical procedures followed by irradiation were used in only 12 cases altogether. All patients were followed for 5 years at least and some up to 20 years or longer.

Some tumors, when first discovered and treated, involved the mid-brain predominantly and others the brain stem. Accordingly an attempt has been made to review such cases in two separate groups. Considering however that no sharp demarcation exists between the two anatomic locations and that both are involved in some cases, we also intend to analyze treatment results in mid-brain and brain stem tumors combined together as though they were a single group (Chart 2 b).

TREATMENT OF MID-BRAIN TUMORS

In the group of 37 patients with mid-brain tumors that we have treated over 5 years ago, histologic diagnosis so far has been obtained in 17 cases. Biopsy material was available in 4 more cases, but the tissue presented to

PLATE 4

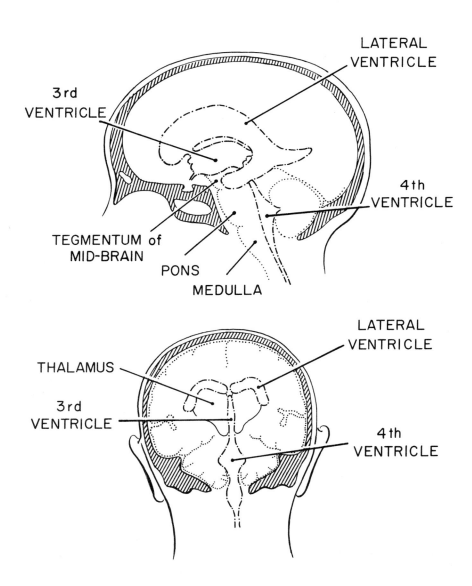

Diagram Illustrating General Topography of Mid-Brain and Pons

neuropathologists was not suitable to arrive at a definite histopathologic diagnosis. The 17 histologically proven mid-brain tumors consist of the following varieties of gliomata: 3 glioblastomas multiforme, 4 unclassified gliomata, 7 astrocytomas, 2 ependymoblastomas and 1 medulloblastoma. Additional histologic proof might come later from patients who are still alive and well at this time.

Postoperative Irradiation

Only 8 of the 37 patients that we have irradiated in the management of their mid-brain tumors have been treated postoperatively. There were 5 patients under 15 years of age and 3 over. All tumors but one have been histologically proven gliomata. Of those 8 patients, 5 have survived over 5 years. Only 2 of these 5 have survived over 10 and 15 years and finally exceeded 20 years of useful life and this without recurrence. These 2 patients were irradiated adequately following partial removal of an unclassified glioma in the one and an ependymoma of the third ventricle in the other.

Irradiation Only, With and Without Surgical Decompressive Procedures

Among the 37 patients who had mid-brain tumors, we have treated a total of 29 only by irradiation. All of them have been followed for at least 5 years from the onset of treatment with radiation. In 12 of these 29 patients, an attempt was made to obtain histologic diagnosis prior to irradiation. Surgical exploration in 7 and needle biopsy in 5 others provided the positive diagnosis desired in only 4 of those 12 cases. One positive biopsy only resulted from the 7 surgical explorations. In final analysis, histologic proof of a primary mid-brain tumor was obtained prior to irradiation in just 4 of the 29 patients, and 3 of the 4 resulted from needle biopsies. At different times subsequent to irradiation, in 6 more cases histologic proof became available through autopsies which revealed different types of gliomata.

Decompressive procedures were accomplished in 18 of the 29 mid-brain tumors treated by irradiation alone. Considering that decompression had to be used in the more critical cases, we believe that such procedures have contributed considerably to our favorable ultimate treatment results by facilitating adequate irradiation. Many patients who were seriously ill and in very poor general condition improved markedly within a few hours to a few days from the time intracranial decompression had been accomplished. Radiation therapy could then be initiated without fear of secondary complications and in particular of aggravating pre-existing cerebral edema. In the few cases in which the effects of intracranial decompression were not so precocious and so definite, the presence of a functioning shunt represented a safeguard which allowed initiation of radiation therapy with confidence, even when the patient was still in a somewhat critical condition.

Decompressive procedures consisted of shunts only in 11 patients, surgical exploration with shunts in 5, and surgical exploration alone in the two remaining ones. No decompressive procedure was used in 11 patients. Of the 12 patients who have survived over 5 years following treatment by irradiation, without surgical removal, 7 had decompression and 5 of these were with shunts alone. This indicates that 39 per cent or 7 of the 18 patients who had intracranial decompression prior to irradiation are among those who have survived 5 years or longer. On the other hand, 45 per cent or 5 of the 11 patients not subjected to decompressive procedures and treated solely by irradiation have survived over 5 years.

It must be emphasized that the length of survival among the 29 patients treated by irradiation alone (Table 5 p. 81), more than 5 years ago, is such that 12 or 41 per cent have survived longer than 5 years. Seven of 17 patients (41 per cent) treated over 10 years ago have exceeded 10 years, whereas 1 of 5 potential survivors has lived over 15 years. There were 2 patients who could have survived 20 years but none did. It appears that in mid-brain tumors treated by irradiation alone, with and without surgical decompressive procedures, the first 2 or 3 years represent the critical period as survival rates begin to level off beyond 3 years (Table 5). The proportion of 5-year survivors seems to be slightly higher (41.0 compared with 37.5 per cent) among those who were irradiated without attempting surgical removal. Five of the 12 were children under 15 years of age.

Life Expectancy and Degree of Recovery

The overall life expectancy of patients with mid-brain tumors treated by adequate irradiation, used alone in 29 cases and postoperatively in 8, is presented in Table 4 on a percentile basis. Our percentages have been derived from the actual survival rates of all the patients whom we have treated for primary intracranial tumors in such anatomic location, with and without histologic diagnoses.

The overall survival rates over 1, 3, 5, 10, 15 and 20 years from the onset of radiation therapy are also illustrated graphically (Chart 2 a) for the 37 patients that we have irradiated as part or all of their treatment for mid-brain tumors. It is estimated that the immediate and long-term results of treatment with adequate irradiation combined with various methods of surgical decompression (18 cases) or partial extirpation (8 cases) or else treated with irradiation alone (11 cases) have indubitably been superior.

Regarding the degree of recovery, the majority of our 37 patients have shown immediate clinical improvement at least temporarily. The long-term quality of survival expressed by the degree of clinical recovery has revealed that 13 of 17 5-year survivors have returned to active useful life. The

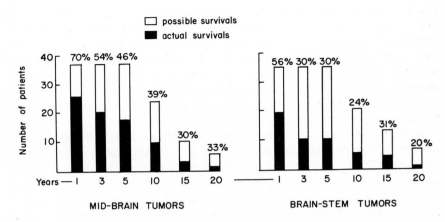

MID-BRAIN AND BRAIN-STEM TUMORS

LIFE EXPECTANCY OF PATIENTS FOLLOWING – IRRADIATION ALONE OR SURGERY PLUS IRRADIATION *

* Irradiation alone in 59 pts. : 29 with mid-brain and 30 with brain-stem tumors

CHART 2 a

Mid-Brain and Brain Stem Tumors—Life Expectancy of Patients Following Irradiation Alone or Operation Plus Irradiation

degree of recovery was fair in 2, and poor in the other 2 patients. The quality of survival has remained good (Grade I) in 9 patients who have survived over 10 years among the 23 treated over 10 years ago. Included in those 9 are 3 survivors of the 10 patients treated over 15 years ago. In turn, the latter group includes 2 of 6 patients, treated over 20 years ago. Each of our long-term survivors has remained in good condition during their survival.

TREATMENT OF BRAIN STEM TUMORS

Philosophy of Treatment Policy

The clinical management of patients with brain stem tumors presents a real challenge to neurologists, neurosurgeons, therapeutic radiologists and other physicians. The anatomic location of pontine tumors in relation to the central nervous system is such that an early diagnosis should be made in the majority of cases. A glioma cannot expand much in the pons without causing symptoms and neurologic signs which can hardly be overlooked.

The prevailing signs of brain stem neoplasms result from the compression or stretching of certain cranial nerves emerging from the pons. The cranial nerve nuclei of the trigeminal, abducent and facial nerves are located in the pons and may be affected directly by tumor growth. The pathways of motor and sensory nerve tracts coming from the mid-brain and cerebellum may be disturbed by neoplastic infiltration in passing through the pons on their way to the medulla. Part of the initial clinical picture may be related in some degree to increased intracranial pressure. In most suspect cases, enlargement of the pons may be demonstrated radiologically by encephalography.

Gliomas of the brain stem, if untreated, may quickly cause irreparable damage to the central nervous system and be rapidly fatal. A prompt decision in relation to treatment is imperative. Having to decide whether to treat palliatively, or not to treat at all and then abandon patients to a fatal outcome is far from being a mere philosophical exercise.

Our present treatment policy regarding patients with brain stem tumors must be clearly stated. We accept to treat by adequate irradiation, without insisting upon histopathologic confirmation of glioma, as such cannot be obtained ordinarily except at the cost of a high mortality rate. We do so providing that firm clinical diagnosis and satisfactory tumor localization are available.

In the period under review, a radical change has occurred at the Montreal Neurological Institute in the management of patients with brain stem tumors. From 1939 to 1947, only 5 patients were treated with radiation, but 2 of these responded to irradiation beyond expectation. In 1947, we began to accept the responsibility of treating by irradiation alone patients presenting indubitable evidence of brain stem tumor, without demanding a histopathologic diagnosis. Since then, we have practised this policy every time that, in consultation with our colleagues in neurosurgery, it was deemed unwise to risk surgical exploration and biopsy or to attempt biopsy by needle aspiration. It may be significant that, from 1947 to 1958 inclusive, we have treated 29 of the 34 patients comprised in our entire series of brain stem tumors irradiated more than 5 years ago.

Morbidity and Prognosis

Pontine tumors consist largely of infiltrative gliomas. Ingraham and Matson[47] believe that all brain stem tumors must be classified as malignant neoplasms, regardless of their specific histology, since their location itself makes them inoperable. They have obtained histological confirmation at operation or at autopsy in 23 of 30 children under 12 years of age. The authors reported that microscopically most pontine tumors consisted of mixed gliomas showing areas of astrocytoma, spongioblastoma polare and glioblastoma multiforme.

Regarding the management of pontine tumors, Ingraham and Matson

(1954) have stated that "surgical exploration for confirmation of diagnosis should be avoided if possible since such surgery is useless". They believe also that the histology of these lesions is not such as to suggest a favorable response to x-ray therapy. The average survival time after onset of symptoms and signs in their series of brain stem tumors has been less than 1 year, regardless of treatment.

The poor prognosis or forecast of the course of brain stem gliomas is a generally recognized and accepted situation which can hardly be remedied. The general consensus appears to be that exploratory and palliative surgical procedures are futile and that radiation therapy is worthless in the care of patients developing gliomas in the pons. In addition to the authors quoted above and many others whose writings could be cited here, Kahn, Bassett, Schneider and Crosby[51] have written that "X-ray therapy is of no avail in the treatment of pontine gliomas and that short-circuiting procedures are useless."

Our experience in the management of patients with brain stem gliomas appears to be worth reviewing. It is based upon the analysis of treatment results after intensive tumor irradiation in some 34 patients observed and followed over 5 to 20 years or longer from the onset of radiation therapy. The evidence presented might bring some revision of thinking. We have been dealing with a group of patients whose prognosis was poor from the time the diagnosis of pontine tumor was made. Therefore patients had nothing to lose and everything to gain in being exposed to a treatment consisting of intensive irradiation primarily.

Presumptive Histologic Diagnosis

Histologic confirmation was available prior to irradiation in only 4 cases in which partial to nearly complete surgical removal had been performed. Biopsies were taken in 3 other cases, but all turned out to be inadequate. A repeat biopsy at the time of tumor reactivation, 15 months following previous surgical exploration and negative biopsy followed by intensive irradiation, revealed a glioblastoma multiforme. Four autopsies also provided late histological confirmation of diagnosis, bringing up to 9 our total of proven cases. These 9 histologically confirmed brain stem tumors consist of the following varieties: 3 glioblastomas, 2 unclassified gliomata, and 4 astrocytomas.

The probability that an expanding lesion in the brain stem be anything but a glioma is relatively minimal. The differential diagnosis lies between pontine gliomas primarily, and possibly syringomyelia or hydromyelia. We know of 2 proven pontine aneurysms.

Results of Treatment by Adequate Irradiation Primarily

Our series comprises 34 cases of brain stem tumors treated more than

5 years ago. Follow-up is complete to this time. Twenty were children ranging from 3 to 15 years of age.

The therapeutic approach in 30 of 34 patients has consisted of intensive irradiation alone, considered adequate for the control of brain stem tumors (Table 5 p. 81). From the onset of radiation therapy, 50 per cent have survived more than 1 year. Of the 15 remaining survivors, 7 lived for 2 or 3 years but in no case did any exceed 36 months. Our analysis reveals that life expectancy is quite good once patients have survived over 3 years without recurrence.

In our series of 30 patients, treated for pontine tumors solely by irradiation, a total of 8 have exceeded the 3- and 5-year survival periods from the time of treatment (Table 5). Five of them (3 under 15 years of age) are still living and well over 9, 15, 16, 19 and 21 years. The remaining 3 5-year survivors, ranging in age between 53 to 64 years, lived 5, 6, and 10 years after treatment. One patient only, among the 8 who survived over 3 and 5 years, ever developed tumor recurrence following initial treatment with radiation alone; he was re-irradiated and improved again for 2 more years. The 6-year survivor died of cancer of the bladder and, at autopsy, presented no evidence of residual tumor nor of postradiation damage in the brain and pons. The third patient died at the age of 74, over 10 years after treatment, without any sign of tumor reactivation.

It appears from our statistical analysis that, unless patients are affected with brain stem tumors in the older age group, 50 to 60 or over occasionally, long-term survivals may be expected in approximately 25 per cent of all patients treated by irradiation alone for brain stem tumors.

Among the 22 patients who manifested clinical evidence of tumor reactivation following a period of clinical improvement exceeding 6 months after irradiation alone, 6 were re-irradiated. They improved again for periods extending from 6 to 24 months, but not one survived over 3 years altogether from the time of initial treatment.

Surgical extirpation was attempted first in 4 patients, 2 adults and 2 children. Their brain stem tumors consisted of one unclassified glioma and 3 astrocytomas. The adults recovered clinically but died of recurrence after 20 and 30 months respectively, despite the addition of adequate postoperative irradiation. The 2 children have now lived 8 and 9 years without recurrence and they are well.

Of the entire group of 34 pontine tumors, 19 survived over one year, in good condition most of the time. It is very gratifying to report that 10 of 34 survived over 5 years, 5 of 21 over 10 years, 4 of 13 over 15 years and 1 over 20 years after treatment (Chart 2a and Table 4 p. 80).

Prognosis in children with brain stem tumors continues to be severe. Only 3 of 20 irradiated under 15 years of age have lived over 3 years following irradiation. All 3 survivors are presently living and well 8, 17, and 21 years after treatment by irradiation alone. There are 2 children whose pontine tumors were extirpated incompletely and irradiated subsequently. That brings long-term survival rates in children up to 22.7 per cent, a total of 5 of 22 patients.

Nearly every patient had immediate clinical improvement for at least 6 to 12 months. The degree of clinical recovery and quality of survival of patients irradiated for brain stem tumors, both under and over 5 years of survival, has been most satisfactory for the major part of life duration following treatment. Among those who have enjoyed long survivals, the quality of living or degree of recovery has been reassessed at the 5-, 10-, 15- and 20-year periods of their living. Every long-term survivor following irradiation for brain stem tumors has remained well, except for one who continued to be totally disabled during the 64 months that she lived after treatment.

The actual survival and recovery rates in our series of 34 patients, predominantly children and young adults, treated for pontine tumors and followed for at least 5 years, clearly point out that life expectancy (Table 4) should no longer be considered so hopeless. This appears to be attributable largely to adequate irradiation (Table 5) and good clinical management. This is illustrated graphically in Chart 2a.

Evaluation of Decompressive Procedures

The beneficial effects of decompression upon the control of gliomas in the management of the brain stem are somewhat difficult to assess. Decompressive surgical procedures have been accomplished in 10 of our 34 patients. The remaining 24 were treated solely by irradiation. Of the 4 patients decompressed at the time of partial removal of their primary tumors, 2 survived over 3 years. Surgical exploration only, without tumor removal, was performed in 2 patients, one of whom is surviving beyond 21 years. Cisterno-ventricular shunts were established in 4 cases prior to irradiation alone and 3 patients are long-term survivors.

Despite contrary opinions, our own experience strongly suggests that surgical decompressive procedures may play a part in the immediate and long-term treatment results of brain stem gliomas. Of 15 patients who lived less than 1 year, with an average survival of 6.6 months, there was only one who had had decompression. Not one of the remaining 9 patients, subjected to some form of surgical decompression before irradiation, lived less than 20 months. It seems significant that among the 10 patients (Chart 2 a) who survived over 5 years after treatment, 6 have had decompression (shunts in 3 of them). It is interesting to note that 4 of those 10 long-term survivors were treated only with radiation. Of 21 treated more than 10 years, 3 of 5 who have survived over 10 years have had decompression. In 13 patients treated over 15 years ago, 2 of the 4 who survived between 15 and 20 years have had decompression. Among the 3 patients who have survived over 20 years after treatment one has had tumor decompression.

COMBINED TREATMENT RESULTS IN MID-BRAIN AND BRAIN STEM TUMORS

The lack of natural anatomic separation between the mid-brain and the pons has been emphasized in the opening section of this chapter. One must also remember that any demarcation between those anatomic regions and the immediate continuing parts of the central nervous system above and below (Plate 4, a and b) is purely conventional. Most tumors found in the mid-brain and brain stem are gliomata ordinarily infiltrative and diffuse in type. These may be expected to extend beyond conventional anatomic boundaries and override one another. We have segregated our tumors either in the mid-brain or else in the brain stem, depending upon the apparent predominance in one location or the other at the outset of their clinical manifestations and signs.

Our clinical material includes several cases in which tumors arising in the mid-brain or in the brain stem were overriding the two anatomic locations, and even extended into the forebrain upwards or into the medulla downwards. Gliomas of the mid-brain and the brain stem have many features in common. Histological confirmation was currently difficult to obtain, so that patients often had to be treated on the basis of a clinical diagnosis only. In either location the prognosis was severe. Their clinical management offered much similarity, since the majority of them were not considered suitable for surgical removal. Most cases in each group were treated by irradiation alone primarily.

In consideration of the above factors and others, we believe it might be interesting to study the overall treatment results by merging mid-brain and brain stem tumors in a single group (Chart 2 b). Of our 71 patients, 59 were treated by irradiation alone primarily, without surgical extirpation. Only 12 were treated surgically first and irradiated afterwards. There were 37 patients with mid-brain and 34 with brain stem glioma treated and followed for more than 5 years, up to 20 and over.

Overall Survival and Recovery Rates

Combined survival rates of the 71 patients that we have treated more than 5 years ago for mid-brain and brain stem tumors are clearly seen over 1, 3, and 5 years respectively (Chart 2 b). Survival rates arising from 44 patients treated over 10 years ago, 23 treated over 15 years and 11 over 20 years, are indicated above the corresponding columns on Chart 2 b.

The long-term recovery rates of mid-brain and brain stem tumors together are most satisfactory. Of the 27 patients who survived over 5 years, 22 (81 per cent) were perfectly well (Grade I) at the 5-year period of their survival, whereas 2 were partially disabled and 3 only were totally

9

AVERAGE RATES FOR BOTH MID-BRAIN AND BRAIN STEM TUMORS
SURVIVALS OVER 1–20 YEARS

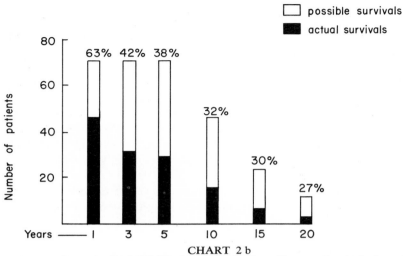

CHART 2 b

Average Rates for Both Mid-Brain and Brain Stem Tumors. Survivals Over 1 to 20 Years

incapacitated. All but 1 of the 14 10-year survivors were well at the end of the 10-year survival period. Those who have survived over 15 and 20 years from onset of irradiation have all enjoyed good useful survival.

RADIATION THERAPY TECHNIQUE

Treatment planning must be individualized to some degree, particularly in relation to the direction of radiation beams and size of fields. In view of the factors just mentioned in the previous paragraphs, we must be fully aware that tumors of the mid-brain may infiltrate not only into the direction of its vertical axis, but also in forward and lateral directions. Necropsy material has shown this in a few cases in which we failed to restrain and control tumor growth by irradiation because such factors were ignored in the planning of treatment.

Treatment fields must therefore be long enough in the vertical axis of the mid-brain and pons to exceed by an adequate margin any probable extension above and below the apparent level of neoplastic infiltration. One posterior and two lateral fields should be used in all cases (Plate 5, a and b). These fields may be narrow (approximately 6 cm. in width) below the level of the foramen magnum. Above that level, because of possible infiltration via the cerebral and cerebellar peduncles, fields must be wide

PLATE 5

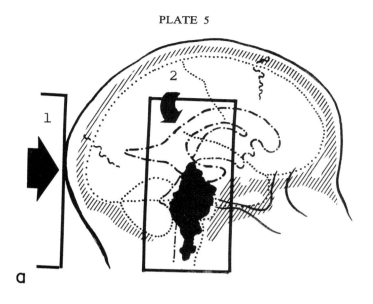

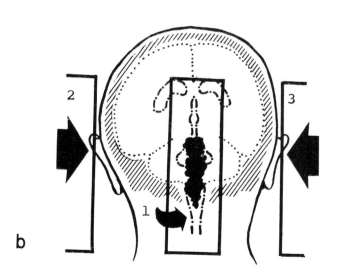

Pontine or Brain Stem Tumor Extending Upward and Downward. Position of Fields and Beam Direction

PLATE 6

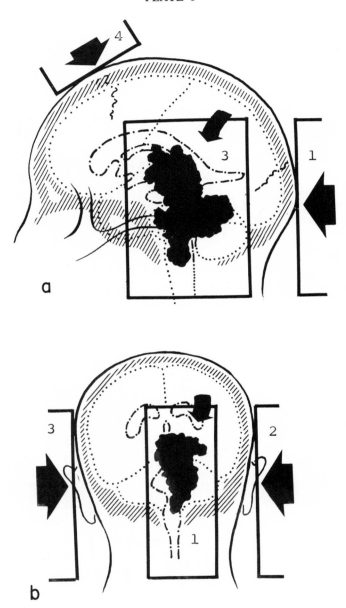

Midline Tumor Extending Superiorly Into the Third Ventricle, Laterally into the Left Cerebral Hemisphere, Posteriorly Into the Cerebellum and Inferiorly Into the Pons and Upper Medulla. Position of Fields and Beam Direction.

PLATE 7

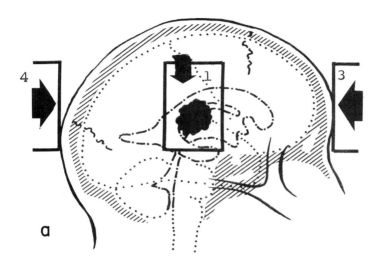

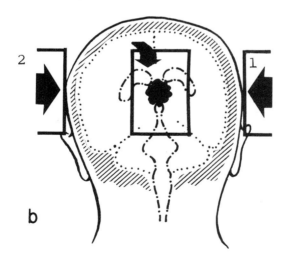

Small Glioma in Upper Posterior Part of Third Ventricle. Position of Fields and Beam Direction

enough to include the posterior part of the third ventricle and the hypo-thalamic region, together with the supratentorial and infratentorial parts of the posterior cranial content.

When mid-brain tumors involve the posterior thalamic and hypothal-amic regions, the anterior limits of gliomatous infiltration may be indefi-nite. Then it is wise to crossfire the tumor-bearing region with an anterior field (Plate 6, a and b), in addition to the other fields just indicated above. Mid-brain and brain stem tumors are not to be pin-pointed with sharply demarcated fields of invariable size or tailored to cover just the apparent area of tumefaction. Gliomata involving those mid-line structures of the central nervous system are nearly always more extensive than they seem to be.

Exceptionally, well-circumscribed small tumors will develop in the posterior and superior regions of the third ventricle. These usually consist of tumors arising from the choroid plexus (cyst or ependymoma) or may represent a pinealoma. Tumors in that anatomic location are generally considered inaccessible for surgical extirpation. Using a small field tech-nique (Plate 7, a and b), we treat such tumors with megavoltage (Co-balt[60]) and tumor doses of 5000 rads in 40 to 45 days.

The mid-brain and pons may have been damaged by the tumor itself and be most vulnerable to irradiation under such conditions. Edema is ordi-narily present to some degree and this must not be increased by irradiation. Against edema corticosteroids may be effective adjuvants, associated with small initial doses of irradiation. Radiation is so far the only therapeutic agent capable of restraining and controlling growth in brain tumors, and it must be administered without exceeding radiation tolerance of the adjacent brain tissue.

Using Cobalt[60], we aim to deliver tumor doses of not less than 5000 rads to the pons and upper medulla, and 6000 rads to the mid-brain region. We treat by irradiation in a single course, on a long protracted basis of 50 to 60 days. In the treatment of mid-brain and brain stem tumors, I would not rely upon smaller doses over shorter periods of time. And that stands despite the consideration that, in principle, the radiobiologic effects on normal brain tissue might be equivalent if a properly reduced time-dose relation were determined and used. We are not convinced that, in practice, such physical modifications might adequately compensate for the increased vulnerability of the adjacent brain tissue being compressed and infiltrated by a glioma growing in the mid-brain or the pons, or both at once.

The important role of the neurosurgeon in providing histologic verifica-tion of the diagnosis, when feasible, and decompression mostly with shunts, is invaluable to patients. The contribution of neurologists, neuroradiolo-gists, nurses and radiological technicians in the overall management of patients treated for mid-brain and pontine tumors is indispensable. Indeed, the results presented here could never have been obtained without superb team work, combined with careful appraisal of the clinical and the radio-biological problems presented by each patient. Radiation per se is not a magic wand.

In conclusion, mid-brain and pontine tumors remain serious neoplastic conditions, but they no longer need to be regarded as hopeless. Patients should not be considered doomed without treatment. Irradiation alone can control the growth of primary gliomata in such critical anatomic locations, providing that a thorough clinical assessment is made in each case in order to plan the volume and extent of intracranial structures to be irradiated adequately. High tumor doses, not exceeding the radiation tolerance of brain tissue must be used, in a single course, protracted over 50 to 60 days. This is the period of time that we consider optimum for adequate irradiation, in consideration of the volume of brain tissue to be irradiated and the fact that adjacent brain tissue is diseased and below normal tolerance.

Surgical procedures should be conservative and be aimed mostly at de-compression and histologic verification, whenever this can be accomplished without unduly risking fatal complication. Mortality associated with ade-quate irradiation alone is most uncommon. Immediate results have been gratifying. More important still are the long-term survival and valid recov-ery rates, observed and reported over 5 to 20 years and longer following irradiation, alone or postoperatively, in mid-brain and brain stem tumors.

Influence of Irradiation on Results of Treatment of Non-gliomatous Primary Intracranial Neoplasms

THE NON-GLIOMATOUS primary intracranial neoplasms comprise a very mixed group. The role of radiation therapy may vary considerably from one type of tumor to another. Intracranial sarcomas represent a rather heterogeneous histologic group of tumors which often respond to radiation therapy better than most would presume. The majority of meningeal tumors can be extirpated completely by surgical removal, so that the number of cases for which radiation therapy is indicated may be rather small. Many of the blood vessel tumors consist of relatively benign hemangiomas which, whether treated or not, may be compatible with a good life expectancy. Hemangioblastomas arising from the cerebellum may be controlled solely by surgical removal in most cases; postoperative irradiation is required only for the few tumors incompletely extirpated. Congenital tumors other than those of vascular origin are few and consist mostly of craniopharyngiomas and chordomas.

Several tumors in our series were diagnosed as pinealomas on clinical basis. In final analysis however, there is not a single histologically proven pinealoma among the non-gliomatous tumors that we have irradiated.

Life Expectancy

In the present series (Table 10) of 70 non-gliomatous intracranial tumors which have been exposed to adequate irradiation, alone or postoperatively, the tabulated results indicate a rather favorable overall life expectancy. All patients were irradiated more than 5 years ago and followed up completely to 1964. There were 46 treated over 10 years ago; 29, over 15 years ago; and 17, over 20 years ago. In 55 or 79 per cent of the 70 cases, irradiation was used postoperatively either because of incomplete surgical removal or else postoperative recurrence (8 meningeal tumors).

Irradiation was used alone (Table 5 p. 81) in the treatment of 15 patients or 21 per cent of the non-gliomatous intracranial neoplasms ir-

136

TABLE 10. Primary Intracranial Neoplasms—Non-gliomatous
Life Expectancy of Patients Treated by
Surgical Removal Plus Irradiation or Irradiation Alone

Types of Tumors	Proportion of Survivals over					
	1 Year	3 Years	5 Years	10 Years	15 Years	20 Years
Sarcomas	11/16	9/16	7/16	4/14	2/5	0/2
Meningeal	24/25	18/25	17/25	11/17	6/10	2/5
Vascular	15/15	15/15	13/15	12/14	8/10	4/7
Congenital	6/8	6/8	5/8	1/4	0/2	0/1
Miscellaneous	5/6	4/6	4/6	4/6	1/2	1/2
All Types	61/70	52/70	46/70	32/45	17/29	7/17

Table drawn up from actual survivors among 70 patients irradiated adequately, 1939 to 1958 inclusive. Clinical follow-up complete to 1964, ranging from a minimum of 5 years up to 25 years. Of the 70 patients, 45 were treated over 10 years ago; 29, over 15 years; and 17, over 20 years. Surgical removal (incomplete) plus post-operative irradiation: 55 patients or 79%. Irradiation alone: 15 or 21%.

radiated more than 5 years ago. In preparing Table 10, we have merely attempted to determine the life expectancy of patients in each category of non-gliomatous intracranial neoplasms which required radiation therapy in our series. Survival rates can be calculated by considering the proportion of those who have survived over 1, 3, 5, 10, 15 and 20 years in relation to the total number of patients irradiated in the management of identical cases. Due to the predominance of meningeal and vascular tumors, which usually carry a favorable prognosis, the proportion of survivals over 5, 10, 15, and 20 years following irradiation is relatively high.

In the non-gliomatous tumors, histologic proof of diagnosis was obtained in 62 of 70 cases or 88.6 per cent. There were 15 patients treated solely by irradiation. The histologic diagnosis has been established in 7 cases, 4 by biopsy and 3 at post mortem.

It is our intention to discuss the influence of irradiation on treatment of non-gliomatous primary intracranial neoplasms. For that purpose, treatment results will be considered by histologic group and according to the tumor location in a few uncommon neoplasms.

INTRACRANIAL SARCOMAS

Malignant tumors may arise intracranially from various tissues of mesenchymal origin and make up the heterogeneous group of sarcomas of the brain. These intracranial sarcomas are not common. Kernohan and Uihlein[56] have made an extensive study of intracranial sarcomas and have found a total of 241 cases, an incidence of 3 per cent in relation to 8070 intracranial tumors.

Histopathologic Complex and Neoplastic Behavior

Intracranial sarcomas comprise tumors of different histopathologic types: fibrosarcomas, reticulum cell sarcomas, perithelial sarcomas, and cerebellar or alveolar sarcomas. Kernohan and Uihlein[56] have included other histological varieties such as giant cell fibrosarcomas, hemangiopericytomas and meningeal sarcomatosis. The anatomic distribution of intracranial sarcomas showed in their series that some 27 per cent involved the cerebellum, and the cerebrum in the balance of the cases. The pons and medulla are rarely affected. The age distribution is quite variable from one series to another. It seems that a high incidence occurs in the first decade consistently.

The prognosis of patients with intracranial sarcomas is less severe than with sarcomatous growths arising in other parts of the body, unless they are diffuse and then invade or replace the brain tissue. Certain intracranial sarcomas originate from the leptomeninges in the posterior cranial fossa and morphologically are practically undistinguishable from medulloblastomas. Zimmerman et al.[123] have reported that cerebellar sarcomas may spread along the subarachnoid spaces just like medulloblastomas and moreover have the ability to metastasize to other parts of the body, outside the central nervous system. Kernohan and Uihlein[56] have made the same observation in relation to intracranial reticuloendothelial cell sarcomas. In our small series, histopathologic evidence (from autopsy) was found that metastases to bone, pleura, peritoneum and abdominal lymph nodes have occurred in 4 cases of cerebellar sarcomas. In one of these cases the peritoneal implant surrounded the end of a ventriculoperitoneal shunt tube. This happened in the only patient in our series who had a shunt established at the time of surgical removal of a primary intracranial sarcoma.

The debated neuropathologic problem of sorting cerebellar sarcomas from medulloblastomas has been discussed in Chapter 5 in the section on the latter tumors. Many neuropathologists have not only expressed the opinion that cerebellar sarcomas are undistinguishable from medulloblastomas, but also believe that all primary malignant tumors should be regarded as a single entity and classified as medulloblastomas. Our present neuropathologists share that viewpoint.

The fact should be emphasized that involvement of the brain from systemic Hodgkin's sarcoma or lymphosarcoma of the small lymphocytic cell type has not been observed by Kernohan and Uihlein[56]. This confirms our personal experience in the management of a substantial number of patients with such lymphomatous sarcomas.

Treatment Results

Our total series of intracranial sarcomas comprises 16 cases: 7 children and 9 adults. In 4 cases the sarcomatous lesions arose from the cerebral hemispheres, whereas in 12 these appeared to originate from the cerebellum or the region of the cerebellopontine angle. The diagnosis of intracranial sarcoma was made at operation at the same time as surgical removal in 14 patients. Intensive irradiation followed surgical treatment in all of them. In the two remaining cases, tissue diagnosis was obtained by needle biopsy and treatment consisted of irradiation only.

There are not enough cases of each histologic variety of primary intracranial sarcoma in our series to report results on such basis. For the same reason, we cannot discuss treatment results in relation to the anatomic location of sarcomas, either supratentorial or infratentorial. The overall survivals in that broad variety of intracranial sarcomas are presented in Table 10. It should be noted that there were only 2 patients treated for more than 20 years, and none have lived that long. There were 2 patients only whom we treated solely by irradiation. These improved dramatically following treatment; nevertheless their tumors recurred, and they lived 18 and 52 months respectively from the onset of treatment.

Our results seem to confirm the opinion of Kernohan and Uihlein that in cases of intracranial sarcoma, radical excision followed by adequate radiation therapy offers a much better chance of prolonging life than in most cases of glioma in similar location and of comparable grade of malignancy. It might be added here that, in our limited experience, adults have survived longer than children.

Recovery rates of patients who have lived over 5, 10, and 15 years after treatment have been satisfactory. Five of the 7 patients who survived over 5 years were perfectly well, whereas 2 were partially disabled when reviewed at that period of time. Of these 5, two were very well over 10 years and one over 15 years. The other 15-year survivor remained partially disabled from the time of treatment.

In discussing medulloblastomas (see page 115), we mentioned that Berger and Elvidge[10] have reported on 20 cerebellar sarcomas and 109 medulloblastomas. One of their objectives was to compare results of treatment between the two groups. Those patients showed an average survival of 4 years and 9 months in cerebellar sarcomas following operation and irradiation, a definitely higher average than in medulloblastomas. Morbidity was less in the 20 patients with cerebellar sarcomas than in the 109 patients with medulloblastomas, since 7 patients with sarcomas or 35 per cent survived over 5 years in comparison with 12 or 11 per cent in the medulloblastoma group.

The reader should be reminded that the only case of postradiation necrosis observed in our entire series of intracranial tumors happened to be a case of cerebellar sarcoma. This case has been discussed in the section on brain necrosis in Chapter 2 (see page 38 and Figs. 4, 5 a and b).

Treatment with radiation focused on the tumor-bearing area was administered to every sarcoma. These malignancies were considered circumscribed lesions for the purpose of treatment planning. Currently, tumor doses equivalent to 6000 rads in 50 to 60 days are delivered, using Cobalt[60] radiation.

It is obvious that the management of intracranial sarcomas is complex because of the variety of histological entities usually comprised in that group of primary intracranial tumors. The majority of workers seem to be of the opinion that, in most histological types, the prognosis is fair. A number of long survivals with good recovery may be expected following surgical removal and adequate irradiation. In the infrequent cases of sarcomatosis arising intracranially and in cerebellar sarcomas which may metastasize outside the central nervous system, irradiation of the entire cerebrospinal axis appears to be indicated. This has become imperative, considering that so many pathologists now agree that cerebellar sarcomas behave like medulloblastomas and in effect should be classified together. Perhaps systemic or intrathecal chemotherapy might be of some value in such cases just as it might be in medulloblastomas.

MENINGEAL TUMORS

Histogenesis and Variety of Histologic Entities

Intracranial tumors arising from the meninges consist in general of slowly growing and sharply circumscribed benign neoplasms. Meningiomas may arise from a variety of tissues of mesenchymal origin. Several histologic entities have been described, mostly in relation to the type of tissue predominating in some meningiomas. Most histologic varieties are benign in character. They grow without ordinarily invading the brain tissue or the adjacent parts of the intracranial content or the cranium itself. Symptoms and clinical signs resulting from meningeal tumors are largely due to pressure and displacement. Many meningiomas are firm and wrapped up in a capsule which is traversed by numerous large blood vessels. These vessels can be of high diagnostic significance when visualized by cerebral angiography.

The histologic diagnosis may consist of meningeal fibromas or fibroblastomas, archnoid fibroblastomas, meningeal or dural endotheliomas, and angiomatous or angioblastic meningiomas. Mixed meningeal tumors have been described. When meningeal neoplasms microscopically appear malignant, the term sarcoma is currently attached to the histological variety. Meningeal sarcomas are usually circumscribed tumors but they may also be diffuse and then invade the brain or the skull. These may occasionally spread extensively, hence the term diffuse sarcomatosis of the meninges. Meningeal tumors located at the base of the skull are often dense and firm, extending en plaque. Zimmerman et al.[123] have emphasized the fact that a same patient may present with several meningiomas.

Incidence

Meningiomas comprise about 15 per cent of all primary intracranial tumors. They occur mostly in middle-aged adults, rarely in children. Zimmerman et al. believe that the prognosis depends more upon the location of meningeal tumors than the histologic appearance. This explains why neurosurgeons tend to classify meningeal tumors according to their anatomic location. The natural history of meningeal tumors is favorable, because their growth is slowly progressive and usually of long duration.

Selection of Treatment: Surgical Extirpation Alone Primarily

The majority of meningeal tumors may be treated successfully by surgical extirpation alone. Surgical results are usually good. Long survivals without recurrence have been reported by many neurosurgeons. Horrax[45] had good survival rates and satisfactory recovery in a large series of patients treated surgically. Among a group of 183 patients, 159 survived operation and 129 of these were followed from 5 to 20 years. Davis and Davis[27] made a follow-up study of 177 patients operated for intracranial meningiomas and reported that 60 patients were alive more than 5 years postoperatively, one being well and active 27 years after operation.

Radiation therapy is not indicated ordinarily after surgical removal of meningiomas. Postoperative irradiation is indicated when the observations made by the neurosurgeon at operation, and the histopathologic evidence obtained are such that certain tumors are properly identified as malignant meningiomas or meningeal sarcomas. In that respect, if a case should be considered borderline, we usually abstain and withhold the use of radiation for later should this ever be needed. Apparently many patients never do need radiation therapy.

The degree of radiosensitivity of malignant meningiomas is variable. This could be predicted merely from the tremendous histological differences in the various types of meningeal tumors. Malignant fibroblastomas have shown a degree of radiosensitivity which varies from moderate to low.

Experience with Postoperative Irradiation When Indicated

Our experience is based upon a group of 25 patients treated ordinarily after operation for malignant meningeal tumors and followed for more than 5 years. Of these 25 patients, 17 were irradiated 10 to 15 days following a first operation. Included among those 17 cases were 2 benign meningiomas that we have irradiated on account of partial removal only. Of the total group of 25, 8 patients were irradiated solely for postoperative recurrences, 3 without another operation and the others after a second or even a third surgical removal. Our overall long-term results (Table 10) strongly suggest that adequate radiation therapy may have a true benficial influence on patients treated for intracranial meningiomas under the conditions stated above.

It is not easy to make a valid objective appraisal of the effects of radiation therapy on meningeal tumors showing malignant characters, either microscopically, or else clinically on account of their invasive behavior. Survival rates are not necessarily a true yardstick, because of the natural tendency of meningeal tumors to grow slowly and to recur infrequently. When they do recur, it is usually many years after surgical extirpation. The ability of patients to recover from the neurologic signs caused by meningiomas should be attributable to surgical removal primarily in most cases in which immediate adequate irradiation is used postoperatively. The degree and duration of recovery may be related to a more complete tumor eradication than estimated, or else might be due to the control by irradiation of actual residual tumor and the resulting prevention of recurrence.

It may be significant that among the 17 patients whom we have irradiated postoperatively as part of their initial treatment, only 2 subsequently developed recurrences of their tumors (a rate of 11 per cent) over periods of observation ranging from 5 to 20 years and over.

Eight of our patients with meningiomas were irradiated only at the time of postoperative recurrence. Of those 8 patients, 3 have recovered and are living over 6, 7, and 17 years without any further recurrence. Three recurrent meningiomas irradiated after their third operation for tumor reactivation improved and survived for an average of 2 years before dying of their disease. The remaining 2 died of unrelated disease 8 and 57 months respectively after irradiation of their recurrent meningioma.

We took the opportunity of observing directly the effect of radiation on a meningeal fibroblastoma which recurred 12 years after initial treatment. The patient was moribund and presented an extensive tumor filling the frontal region, eroding the base of the skull, invading the right nasal cavity and bulging through the right orbit with the eye down on the cheek (fig. 8 a, b). The patient was treated with kilovoltage radiation and received a total tumor dose of 6500 rads in 60 days. His clinical condition improved slowly, as the neoplastic manifestations gradually regressed to a considerable degree. (Fig. 8c, d) He completed his treatment as an out-patient and survived 2 years in good condition before further recurrence and final episode. The clinical evidence in this hopeless case has clearly demonstrated that adequate radiation therapy may be of definite value in the management of meningeal fibroblastomas.

It seems reasonable to consider that the low recurrence rate (11 per

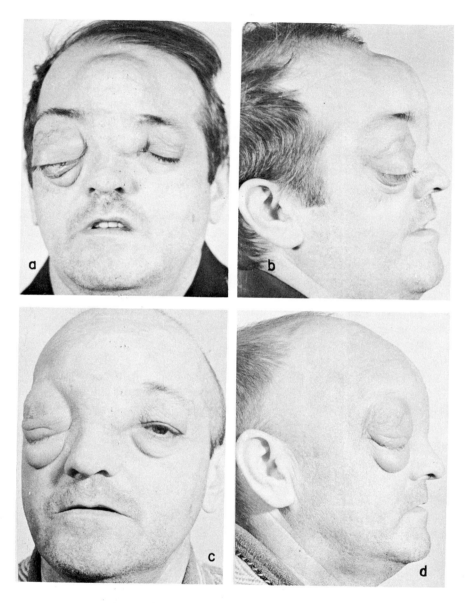

Figures 8 a and b, Recurrent meningeal fibroblastoma bulging under the skin after breaking through the frontal, nasal and orbital bones. Patients was moribund. (See case report.)

c and d, Follow-up pictures, 4 months after onset of course of x-ray therapy with average tumor dose of 6500 rads in 60 days. With marked tumor regression, the patient made a dramatic clinical recovery, physically and mentally, during initial 3 to 4 weeks of treatment

cent) in our small series (17 immediate postoperative cases) represents objective evidence that radiation therapy plays a useful role in the combined treatment of malignant meningeal tumors by surgical extirpation and irradiation. Further evidence may be derived from the clinical improvement and long survivals, without additional recurrence, that we have observed in several patients irradiated only when they manifested postoperative recurrences.

The quality of survival, based upon the degree of clinical recovery experienced by the patients, has been reviewed. This has revealed that, of the 17 patients who have lived longer than 5 years, 14 are still living and in excellent condition from 5 to 20 years and longer after treatment. The only exception is a man who has remained partially disabled since onset of treatment 13 years ago.

Of 3 who died over 5 years after treatment, one was alive and well for 18 years until he died of unrelated disease; another died of recurrence after 12 years of survival with partial disability; and a third one was disabled during the 5 years that he survived.

Doses approaching the normal brain tolerance must be administered. When malignant meningiomas are irradiated, tumor doses equivalent to 6000 to 6500 rads in 50 to 60 days should be administered with megavoltage (Cobalt[60]) radiation. Crossfiring technique with four fields may be adequate. Wedge filter technique may be more suitable in selected cases.

In conclusion, our experience in this center, like in many others, is that treatment of most of intracranial meningiomas is primarily and essentially a surgical problem. The role of radiation therapy in the management of these tumors should be limited to postoperative irradiation of the meningiomas considered malignant by neurosurgeons at the time of operation and subsequently by the neuropathologists. Irradiation is particularly indicated postoperatively when surgical removal is considered incomplete. Radiation therapy has proved to be beneficial in the treatment of postoperative recurrence of meningiomas.

INTRACRANIAL VASCULAR TUMORS

Intracranial expanding lesions of vascular origin consist essentially of two separate pathologic entities: cerebral angiomas which represent congenital malformations, and hemangioblastomas that are true neoplastic lesions.

Our overall experience in radiation therapy applied to the management of such blood vessel lesions rests upon 9 cerebral angiomas and 6 hemangioblastomas, followed over 5 years up to 20 and longer.

CEREBRAL ANGIOMAS

Intracranial angiomas are classified with tumors merely because they are space-occupying lesions. These are not new growths inasmuch as histogenesis is concerned. Cerebral angiomas are vascular anomalies representing congenital malformations which involve arteries and veins and their ramifications principally. Intracranial angiomas are supratentorial lesions located almost exclusively in the cerebral hemispheres, rarely in the cerebellum. Such lesions may be present for years without clinical manifestation of their existence. The discovery of unsuspected and asymptomatic angiomatous anomalies may be fortuitous on the occasion of cerebral angiography.

Low Morbidity

When cerebral angiomas ever cause clinical evidence leading to their discovery, this occurs predominantly in the third or fourth decades of life, and even later. Cerebral angiomas rarely manifest themselves during infancy and childhood. Our youngest patient was 17 years of age. Cerebral angiomas may manifest themselves when they affect the adjacent cerebral tissue to the extent of causing symptoms, with or without neurologic signs. The occasion for that is sometimes a slow leak from blood vessels or else a spontaneous hemorrhage of some degree. These lesions seldom endanger a patient's life, so that survival rates may not be an indication of the effectiveness of a therapeutic method employed.

Indication for Treatment and Selection of Therapeutic Methods

Cerebral angiomas should be considered for treatment only when such vascular lesions are producing symptoms. The treatment of angiomas of the brain, when located close to the surface of a cerebral hemisphere, may consist of surgical extirpation of the lesion providing this is situated well beyond the motor cortex or other critical area. If a cerebral angioma happens to be deeply located in one hemisphere, the ligation of a major feeding vessel might be contemplated and prove to be feasible.

The majority of deeply seated cerebral angiomas should be managed conservatively. Such cases represent a valid indication for adequate radiation therapy. The radiobiologic objective is to induce in the tumor capillaries and venules primarily a reaction of vascular occlusion or endarteritis obliterans. Such vascular effect may progress slowly and eventually result, 2 to 3 years and perhaps longer after treatment, in the direct or secondary occlusion of a number of medium sized and some larger thin walled blood vessels in the area involved. The clinical outcome for patients should be relief in symptoms and cessation of repeated episodes of bleeding or even moderate hemorrhaging. In some cases, even though the condition may seem to be clinically arrested, radiation therapy may not bring correction of the neurologic deficit caused by the vascular lesion.

We have previously[15] suggested that a tumor dose of 3500 rads over a period of 30 to 35 days should be adequate to induce the desired radiobiologic effects. With Cobalt[60] high energy radiation, tumor doses of 4000 to 4500 rads over the same period of time are recommended.

Treatment Results

Our experience in the management of cerebral angiomas, treated and followed for more than 5 years, comprises 9 cases only. There were 7 patients actively treated by irradiation alone. Included among these 7 were 2 patients who had surgical exploration and decompression, but without any direct attempt at surgical extirpation of the lesion itself. Of the total of 9 patients, 2 were treated surgically first and irradiated subsequently because of incomplete removal of the angiomatous blood vessels. One of these 2 patients had the only cerebellar angioma that we have treated.

Survivals range from 12 to 24 years, except for 1 patient who died from bronchogenic carcinoma. The latter patient had an autopsy which revealed that angiomatous blood vessels were still present in the right parietooccipital region. Two patients died of unrelated disease. In this series of 9, the remaining 6 patients are still living and well, all being practically symptom-free.

Objective evidence of results of radiation therapy in cerebral angiomas is not frequently available. Assessment by arteriography would be desirable, perhaps 2 years or longer after treatment, and again approximately 3 years later. A follow-up angiogram is not easy to obtain on the part of the patients and others concerned.

Not included in this series is the case of a patient with a deep cerebral angioma treated over 2 years ago with radiation alone. His lesion received, in a single course, a tumor dose of 4000 rads over a period of 35 days. Clinically he has been well and symptom-free for over 2 years. Follow-up angiograms were made 1 and 2 years respectively after the onset of radiation therapy. As yet, these radiologic studies have not shown conclusive evidence of vascular occlusion and obliteration.

On one occasion only, at a meeting, I have seen a case in which follow-up angiograms, made some 2 years after radiation therapy, demonstrated apparent disappearance of smaller as well as larger angiomatous vessels which could no longer be visualized. Such changes might have been related to postirradiation endarteritis obliterans or else to vascular thrombosis due to some other factor such as hemorrhage within the region involved.

Objective evaluation of the degree of recovery from cerebral angioma is not simple. Subjective appreciation has to be accepted on the basis of symptomatic relief. In that respect, it appears from our follow-up observations that radiation therapy may have had some beneficial influence. Radiation therapy alone is particularly indicated for patients presenting evidence of repeated small hemorrhages in the affected vascular territory.

HEMANGIOBLASTOMAS

True Neoplastic Nature and Incidence

Hemangioblastomas are vascular tumors considered true neoplastic lesions. They arise from the cerebellar hemispheres almost exclusively. Hemangioblastomas, being of low grade malignancy, usually are well-demarcated tumors developing slowly in the infratentorial region. With the majority of cerebellar astrocytomas, hemangioblastomas share the characteristic of growing within a cyst where they form a solid nodule attached to some part of the cyst wall. Histologically, these neoplastic formations contain abundant capillaries with strands of endothelial cells lying between them and more or less cystic vascular spaces filled with blood.

The diagnosis of hemangioblastoma may be suspected but can be made at operation only, when the cyst is opened and the neoplasm deflated after the blood supply is interrupted. Confirmation of diagnosis will have to await microscopic examination of tumor tissue. The incidence of these vascular tumors is low, less than 1 per cent of all intracranial neoplasms.

Hemangioendothelioma is a histologic variant. The basic cell is also endothelial in origin and appears to participate in the proliferation of capillaries, more or less invasive in character, together with the formation of nodular tumor masses in the periphery of the cysts.

Treatment Primarily Surgical

Complete surgical removal of hemangioblastomas can be accomplished successfully in a high proportion of cases. Horrax[45] reported on 48 patients, 41 of whom survived postoperatively. Four of these had local manifestations of Hippel-Lindau's disease. Thirty-five, or 81.3 per cent of the 41 patients who survived operation, have lived between 5 to 20 years and were able to engage in useful activities.

Combined Treatment with Postoperative Irradiation

Irradiation is indicated postoperatively as part of the treatment of hemangioblastomas when these cannot be removed completely. Radiation therapy must be administered in all cases exhibiting malignant characters.

The malignant nature of hemangioblastomas may be demonstrated at operation by the infiltrative character of the neoplastic process which prevents total extirpation of the tumor, or else may be revealed subsequently by the microscopic findings. Postoperative recurrences may be treated by irradiation. Davis and Davis[27] suggest that radiation therapy should be used routinely in the management of hemangioblastoma and can be of great benefit.

In this group of intracranial vascular tumors, our series comprises 6 cases followed for more than 5 years: 4 hemangioblastomas and 2 hemangioendotheliomas, all located in the cerebellar region except for 1 cerebral hemangioblastoma. Partial surgical extirpation of tumor was accomplished in 5 patients. Treatment was completed by postoperative irradiation. The sixth patient was subjected to surgical exploration, but tumor removal was considered unwise because the neoplasm extended into the medulla. The tissue obtained by biopsy was not adequate for confirmation, by microscopic studies, of the gross diagnosis of hemangioblastoma made by the surgeon at operation. In this case, active treatment consisted of surgical decompression and irradiation alone.

Results of combined treatment show that only one of our 6 patients died of hemangioblastoma. This happened during a second operation performed because of tumor recurrence, 51 months after surgical exploration and irradiation. A patient died of unrelated disease 16 years after incomplete surgical removal and intensive irradiation of a histologically verified hemangioendothelioma; at autopsy, no evidence of residual tumor was found. His tumor had received 5000 rads in 40 days. The remaining 4 patients are still living 10, 14, 20 and 23 years after combined treatment.

Regarding the quality of survival over the years, 3 of our long-term survivors continue to be in excellent condition. The remaining survivor (over 10 years) is partially disabled, not working, but able to care for himself. This patient is the one mentioned above who had surgical exploration without tumor removal, and effectively is our only case of hemangioblastoma treated by irradiation alone. The patient, who died of unrelated disease 16 years after treatement, had never recovered completely; he remained ataxic and non-employable during his entire survival.

Because of the potential malignant character of hemangioblastomas, tumor doses varying between 3000 and 5000 rads in 35 to 50 days have been administered with kilovoltage radiation. Hemangioendotheliomas are considered more malignant in character, and tumor doses of 5000 to 6000 rads have been given over periods of 45 to 50 days. Now that megavoltage is readily available, Cobalt[60] radiation or its equivalent, or higher energy radiation, should be used in the treatment of those tumors, aiming at the maximal tumor doses just mentioned.

In conclusion, treatment of hemangioblastomas and hemangioendotheliomas is primarily a surgical problem. Long-term survival rates following surgical treatment alone (Horrax, 83 per cent) have been most gratifying, as the quality of survivals was good and the incidence of recurrence low.

From our limited experience in the treatment of tumors in the hemangioblastoma group, it seems that surgical removal combined with postoperative irradiation may be beneficial to selected patients. Adequate irradiation may have contributed to growth restraint and prevention of recurrence of residual tumors, some relatively benign and others definitely malignant in character. In that respect, long survivals and lasting good recoveries may be attributable to the combined surgical and radiologic therapeutic approach in the clinical cases that we have reviewed.

CONGENITAL TUMORS

There are several types of primary intracranial expanding lesions which are considered congenital in origin. Those of vascular structure, like cerebral angiomas, have been discussed already. Craniopharyngiomas are the most frequently found neoplasms of congenital nature. Chordomas are infrequent.

CRANIOPHARYNGIOMAS

Nomenclature and Pathologic Characteristics

Craniopharyngiomas are histologically benign intracranial tumors, considered malignant on account of their location and their natural behavior. They induce severe pathologic disturbances often difficult to control. The majority of craniopharyngiomas are found above the sella turcica. Others may arise within the sella itself. Infrequently, such tumors may be found in the roof of the pharynx.

The term craniopharyngioma was coined by Cushing. It includes a variety of tumors of the same origin but different nomenclature: suprasellar cysts, hypophyseal duct tumors, craniopharyngeal duct cysts, Rathke's pouch tumors, and adamantinomas.

Craniopharyngiomas designate all intracranial growths that arise in the hypophyseal region and are composed of cystic formations. Characteristically, these cystic cavities are lined with squamous epithelium and filled with pale yellow oily fluid, the latter containing cellular debris and cholesterol crystals. Craniopharyngiomas may be solid and consist of squamous epithelium.

The incidence of craniopharyngiomas varies between 2 and 4 per cent in large series of intracranial tumors. These tumors occur most frequently in children and young adolescents who present clinical evidence of adiposo-genitalis or Fröhlich's syndrome. Craniopharyngiomas may also be found in adults in whom they often simulate chromophobe adenomas or suprasellar meningiomas. Symptoms are those resulting from pituitary suppression or compression of other adjacent structures in particular the optic chiasm and the floor of the third ventricle.

Inherent Treatment Difficulties

In view of the cystic component present in the majority of craniopharyngiomas, the ideal treatment would consist of craniotomy, emptying of the cystic cavity and surgical extirpation of the entire cyst wall. This may be a hazardous procedure to perform in that anatomic location, because of the vicinity of highly vulnerable structures. Solid tumors, in principle, could be extirpated. In practice, this is difficult to accomplish in toto without serious complications.

Combined Surgical and Radiologic Treatment

In recent years, Kramer, McKissock and Concannon[60] have recommended that patients with craniopharyngiomas be subjected to combined surgical removal and postoperative intensive irradiation. Their experience seems to indicate that such combined treatment is likely to produce the best results. Of 10 patients treated in that fashion, 9 were alive and well for over 6 years after treatment. None of them were showing any evidence of damage to the brain as result of irradiation. Kramer *et al.* have suggested that surgery be limited to the minimum necessary to prove the diagnosis and evacuate the cyst. The rest of the treatment should consist of high energy radiation delivered by external beams, carefully directed to the tumor. They have used doses varying in children from 5000 rads in 37 days to 6500 rads in 57 days, and in adults from 5580 rads in 39 days to 6950 rads in 51 days.

The author's material comprises only 4 cases of craniopharyngiomas treated for more than 5 years. There were 3 children under 15 years of age and 1 adult. A young boy of 5 years of age was treated 11 years ago by fluid aspiration of a large multiloculated cyst and external irradiation to a tumor dose of 2200 rads in 28 days. He returned 9 months later when the cyst had to be aspirated again. Subsequently he remained symptom-free for more than 5 years. He then returned once more on account of clinical evidence of refilling of the cyst. Following further fluid aspiration, radioactive colloidal gold was injected into the cavity of the cyst in an attempt to prevent further fluid formation and accumulation. This was not successful, and 6 months later a large portion of the cyst was removed surgically. At the time of this report the patient is now a young man who is symptom-free

11 years following initial treatment. In the light of the experience of Kramer *et al.* it seems that the dose of radiation administered by us was probably not high enough to induce lasting results.

The other 2 children in our series of craniopharyngiomas were treated by surgical removal and intensive postoperative irradiation; the tumor doses exceeded 5000 rads in 45 and 50 days respectively. Both children are alive and well at this time, 5 and 6 years after treatment. Our fourth patient was an adult whose clinical condition improved following similar treatment. He was well for 5 years, but has been disabled for the subsequent 2 years of his life since he went blind and developed an ascending paraplegia.

The management of craniopharyngiomas should be reconsidered. It appears that treatment by conservative surgical methods combined with adequate doses of radiation, as proposed by Kramer and associates, might offer patients the best chance of lasting results and good recovery with minimal treatment morbidity. Since craniopharyngiomas occur predominantly in children, it will be interesting to observe what the future will hold for them and to what extent long-term follow-up data may reveal prolonged control of such tumors without reactivation.

INTRACRANIAL CHORDOMAS

Pathology and Natural Behavior

Chordomas are congenital tumors originating from embryonic rests of the notochord. These neoplasms may be found anywhere along the vertebral column, but occur predominantly at the base of the skull and in the sacrococcygeal region.

Intracranial chordomas are not frequent. Such tumors arise ordinarily from the posterior region of the basisphenoid, below the dorsum sellae, at level of the clivus. Chordomas may bulge posteriorly within the base of the cranial cavity where they stretch the basilar artery and press upon the pons. These tumors may also extend upward through the sella turcica and compress the pituitary gland before emerging above the sella. From there, chordomas may expand in the hypothalamic region, more or less in a spherical fashion, and induce pressure symptoms by involvement of the adjacent structures. At times, chordomas developing from the basisphenoid will erode the base of the skull, invade the sphenoidal sinuses and finally break into the nasopharynx.

Histologically, chordomas can be identified readily. Microscopic examination of tumor sections shows a histologic structure resembling tissue of the embryonic notochord. Mitotic figures are scanty. These neoplasms are considered malignant not so much on account of their histopathologic appearance but because of their tendency to invade and destroy bone, soft tissue and brain. For these reasons, chordomas are virtually impossible to eradicate and tend to regrow rapidly after surgical removal, whether or not irradiation has been added to the treatment postoperatively. Intracranial chordomas do not tend to metastasize, and when they do this is ordinarily a late occurrence.

Treatment Reports in Current Literature

Dyke and Davidoff[30] were of the opinion that radiation therapy for the most part is not satisfactory in the management of intracranial chordomas. These authors have expressed their firm belief that the response of chordomas to radiation is unpredictable, and that all cases should be irradiated postoperatively.

Wood and Himadi[120] reviewed 16 cases of chordomas of which 7 were intracranial. Two of their patients treated by partial surgical removal and irradiation survived over 5 years from the time of treatment. One of these survived more than 9 years following biopsy and irradiation to a tumor dose of 8000 r. They expressed the view that the ultimate prognosis of patients with intracranial chordomas is poor. It is doubtful that a case has ever been cured permanently. In their opinion a 5-year survival is no criterion of cure, as many chordomas grow slowly and metastasize late.

A study of 59 cases of chordomas was presented by Dahlin and Mc Carty.[25] Fifteen of their cases arose intracranially from the region of the clivus, one of these being an autopsy finding. They stated that the results of treatment of spheno-occipital chordomas have been discouraging in most instances. Only 1 of the 14 patients treated for intracranial chordoma survived more than 5 years. They believe that radiation therapy did not seem to alter appreciably the course of the disease in the patients on whom it was employed. Details of radiation treatment are not mentioned.

Recently, Kamerin, Potanos and Pool[52] have reported a series of 30 chordomas of which 16 were intracranial. It is interesting to note that a retropharyngeal mass was present in 5 of their 16 cases. Radiographic examination demonstrated bone destruction in the region of the sella turcica in 13 patients. In the management of intracranial chordomas, Kamerin et al. believe that a tissue diagnosis can be established by pharyngeal or sphenoid sinus biopsy. Operation would be indicated only for decompression purposes or to ascertain the diagnosis. This should be followed by intensive radiation therapy. Tumor doses of 5000 r or more are recommended. Eleven patients have been followed for longer than 1 year, and in 7 of them recurrences were observed approximately 1 year after treatment. Five patients have survived over 5 years from the time of treatment, the longest survivals being 11 and 14 years. Kamerin et al. observed only 1 case of distant metastasis and this was in the lungs. Of their 16 patients treated for intracranial chordomas, 6 were able to return to normal activity but no patient was thought to be free of tumor.

Value of Combined Surgical and Radiologic Treatment

Our experience with intracranial chordomas consists of 4 histologically verified cases. Three patients who had partial removals combined with postoperative irradiation survived 2, 10 and 36 months respectively. The remaining patient survived nearly 6 years. She had been treated with radiation alone on the basis of a clinical diagnosis of chromophobe adenoma. This patient was well for over 5 years but remained blind in her right eye. She was admitted with a tumor bulging in the nasopharynx 1 month before she died of massive hemorrhage. Autopsy revealed a chordoma.

Intracranial chordomas clinically behave like highly malignant tumors from the time they are discovered and the diagnosis is firmly established. There is general agreement that the majority of these tumors carry a bad prognosis.

The role of surgical procedures is mainly to assist in obtaining a tissue diagnosis rather than contribute to tumor control. The evidence presented above indicates that chordomas are rather radioresistant even to high doses of radiation. However, radiation therapy seems capable of inducing some degree of growth restraint and palliation of symptoms. An aggregate of the 41 intracranial chordomas reported in the above series shows that a total of 9 patients have lived more than 5 years from the onset of treatment, suggesting that a 5-year survival rate of approximately 22 per cent may be expected following a combined treatment.

Doses approaching the normal brain tolerance must be administered. When malignant chordomas are irradiated, tumor doses equivalent to 6000 to 6500 rads in 50 to 60 days should be administered with megavoltage (Cobalt^{60}) radiation. Crossfiring technique with four fields may be adequate.

If prolongation of life among the patients who have had long survivals may be partly attributable to postoperative irradiation, radiation therapy should be used in the management of all cases of intracranial chordomas for whatever beneficial effect it might achieve.

PINEALOMAS

Pathogenesis and Incidence

Pinealomas are tumors originating from the parenchyma of the pineal gland. Other terminology consists of pineal dysgerminoma and chorioma. It seems that pinealomas are no longer considered as gliomatous tumors.

Zimmerman *et al.*[123] believe that pinealomas represent teratomatous neoplasms of congenital origin. In their experience many of these tumors do not even involve the pineal body but are found along the base of the brain as in the tuber cinereum and the chiasmal region. Pinealomas are considered by some as the prevalent tumors involving the posterior part of the third ventricle.

Other tumors in the same location (cysts of the choroid plexus or ependymomas) may resemble and mimic pinealomas. These pineal neoplastic lesions are locally invasive in character and often cause obstruction of the aqueduct of Sylvius with secondary damage in the brain. Occasionally pinealomas may spread along the cerebrospinal pathways.

The true incidence of pinealomas is difficult to determine. Zimmerman *et al.*[123] had 6 cases out of 335 primary intracranial tumors. Cushing[123] had 16 out of 2209, and Zulch *et al.*[127] had 25 in 6000 tumors. It appears that the incidence derived from large series of intracranial neoplasms varies between 0.5 and 2.0 per cent. Pineal tumors occur mostly in children or young adults and may be associated with pubertas praecox.

Treatment with Shunts and Irradiation Alone

Because of the high operative mortality associated with attempts at surgical removal, microscopic verification is not obtained very often. In general, surgical removal of pinealomas is not done and the treatment consists of shunts plus external radiation therapy. Pinealomas are said to be radiosensitive and capable of giving a high percentage of long survivals.

I have seen only one proven pinealoma and this is not included in the present series since it has to be considered untreated. The patient was a child aged 14 who had been accepted for treatment by irradiation alone with a presumptive diagnosis of pinealoma. A ventriculoperitoneal shunt had been established prior to initiation of x-ray treatment. He died of meningitis a few days after the onset of radiation therapy. At autopsy, apart from meningitis, a teratoma of the pineal gland was found.

Scarceness of Proven Pinealomas for Treatment Evaluation

Our series comprises 5 cases in which a clinical or presumptive diagnosis of pinealoma was made. These cases have been classed in the group of midbrain tumors. One patient died 6 months after adequate radiation therapy and, at autopsy, the suspected pinealoma proved to be a glioblastoma multiforme. The other 4 patients were also treated with irradiation alone, without histologic confirmation of diagnosis. All 4 are living and well, 2 of them 6 years after treatment and the other 2 over 10 years. A similar situation seems to be prevailing in most reports that I have found. Patients are being treated on presumptive diagnoses but histological verifications are generally lacking.

Personally, I am unable to assess the value of irradiation in treating pinealomas for lack of accurate data, both from my own clinical material or from the current literature. Brain tumors, which are presumed to be pinealomas, have been treated empirically, by crossfiring method using small beams of Cobalt[60] radiation, aiming at tumor doses of 5000 rads over 40 to 45 days (Plate 7, a and b).

MISCELLANEOUS AND UNDETERMINED INTRACRANIAL TUMORS

In every series of primary intracranial neoplasms there must be a small group comprising miscellaneous histologically verified tumors. Our series includes 1 heterotopic cyst partially removed, a perineurial fibroblastoma, and a paraganglioma. All 3 patients were treated by combined surgical removal and postoperative irradiation. These patients are presently living 24, 12 and 10 years respectively from the onset of irradiation.

Despite clinical evidence and objective findings convincing enough to justify surgical exploration and subsequent irradiation, the diagnosis of brain tumor has remained undetermined in 3 cases. These patients were subjected to craniotomy for expanding lesions that could not be identified at operation and therefore not extirpated; attempts at biopsy turned out to be negative. Two of the patients so treated, as though they had histologically proven brain tumors, died with all the signs of intracranial tumors 6 months and 2 years respectively following irradiation alone. The third patient has recovered and is alive and well over 10 years after the onset of radiation therapy.

Results in Children Irradiated under the Age of 15 Years for Brain Tumors

IN VIEW of the potential late repercussions which might occur and affect the mental development and somatic growth of children irradiated for brain tumors, it is imperative that every aspect of this problem be thoroughly scrutinized. Considerable apprehension exists concerning the exposure to ionizing radiation of the brain and skull of children. Many are fearful that irradiation of the central nervous system during infancy and childhood might interfere with its anatomic and physiologic development in the latter period of its natural evolution. The central nervous system is believed to reach its maturity about the age of 15. There is a strong and persistent belief that the pituitary gland may be affected adversely by direct or indirect exposure to radiation during treatment of brain tumors in children, and that serious disturbance might result in somatic growth and other endocrine functions.

Radiation therapy of brain tumors in children is considered hazardous by many. Although it might seem that way, when one ponders the tumor doses actually used over the last 25 years in the children that we irradiated for brain tumors, we believe that the results of such therapy fully justify its application. In our opinion, the magnitude of the tumor doses used is required for treatment to be adequate and control malignant tumors that will inevitably destroy the brains of children and take their lives away as well. It is unjustifiable to allow brain tumors to become so harmful and lethal, for fear of some potential risks of radiation exposure. Radiation hazards in such cases are remote and hypothetical, in contrast with brain tumor risks which are immediate and real.

Over the years, the continued observation of our cases, through periodic follow-up examinations, has allowed us to make some evaluation of the effects of irradiation of the central nervous system in the young. The usefulness and relative safety of intensive ionizing radiation therapy in the management of intracranial neoplasms in children can be evaluated best by

156

analysis of the results observed during the first few months or even years after treatment and also by study of long-term recovery and survival rates.

SALIENT FACTS REGARDING BRAIN TUMORS IN CHILDREN

Incidence of Brain Tumors in Children in Relation to Malignancies

Our total experience is based upon 119 children of ages ranging from a few months to 15 years at the time of irradiation of their skull and intracranial content in the management of their tumors. This represents 21 per cent of the 564 patients whom we have irradiated for primary intracranial neoplasms over a 20-year period, 1939 to 1958 inclusive, and followed ever since treatment. This incidence rate is in keeping with the rates reported by other authors. It is of interest to note that the incidence of primary brain tumors represents approximately 12 per cent of all malignancies in children aged 15 or under. In that respect brain tumors occupy the second rank, coming just after leukemia. The overall age distribution in our series is also identical to the pattern reported by others. Brain tumors are rare in the first year of life, gradually increase in frequency to reach their peak incidence between the ages of 6 and 10, and then decrease to the incidence level attained at 5 years.

Predominance and Low Incidence of Certain Categories of Primary Brain Tumors

The classification of our material has been made according either to the histologic type of primary neoplasms or to their location in the mid-brain and brain stem (Table 11). Histologic verification is complete in 98 of 119

TABLE 11. Primary Brain Tumors Irradiated in Children*

	Children in Series		5-Year Survivors	
	No.	Per Cent	No.	Per Cent
Gliomata				
Glioblastoma	3	2	3	—
Glioma, unclassified	11	9	4	36
Astrocytoma	16	14	12	75
Ependymoma	7	6	5	71
Medulloblastoma	37	31	10	27
Mid-brain	14	12	8	57
Brain stem	20	17	5	25
Non-gliomatous tumors				
Sarcoma	7	6	2	28
Craniopharyngioma	3	2	3	100
Meningeal fibroblastoma	1	1	1	100
	119	100%	50	42%

* All children were treated under 15 years of age, 78 postoperatively and 41 with irradiation alone—1939 to 1958.
Clinical follow-up complete to 1964.

children or practically 80 per cent of the cases. In our series of children irradiated in the treatment of primary intracranial neoplasms, only 11 of 119 or 9 per cent were treated for non-gliomatous neoplasms.

Certain histological types are rare in children. In our series there are no blood vessel tumors, and just one malignant meningioma. Ingraham and Matson[47], in a series of 313 intracranial tumors in children under 12 years of age, had 9 hemangiomas and 1 meningioma, and no cerebellar hemangioblastoma nor pinealoma. In the glial group of tumors, oligo-dendrogliomas are infrequent and there are none in our series. Only 3 glioblastomas multiforme are listed, all 3 being hemispheral tumors, but there were 4 more glioblastomas found in areas in which our primary intracranial gliomas were classed by anatomic location rather than by histologic group.

The predominant categories of gliomas in our series of children are by far the medulloblastomas, followed by mid-brain and brain stem tumors, astrocytomas, and others (Table 11). In regards to astrocytomas, one half or 8 cases were cerebellar tumors irradiated because of incomplete re-moval, whereas the other 8 were cerebral tumors. Astrocytomas identified (3 cases) in the mid-brain and the brain stem are not included among the astrocytomas classified by histologic group.

It is well known that brain tumors occurring in children arise predomi-nantly from the infratentorial region. In a series of 273 children with brain tumors, French[37] has reported that 48 per cent were supratentorial and 52 per cent infratentorial. Ten per cent in his series consisted of glioblas-tomas. Glioblastomas are less frequent in children than in adults. Accord-ing to French, when they do occur in children, approximately 50 per cent of them are located in the brain stem.

INDICATIONS FOR TREATMENT AND SELECTION OF METHOD

All children with the diagnosis of primary intracranial tumor were not subjected to radiation therapy. Indications and contraindications for ir-radiation have been determined upon the basis outlined above (Chapter 3). These are the same for children as for adults. In many instances, children were accepted for treatment despite their critical condition, and yet several eventually recovered. Some of our long-term survivals belong to this group of cases.

The majority (66 per cent) of children have been treated by surgery followed with intensive irradiation, usually initiated 2 or 3 weeks after operation. Actually, 78 of the 119 children were treated by surgical re-moval followed by intensive irradiation. Irradiation was the sole thera-peutic agent applied directly for the control of tumor growth in 41 (34 per cent) of the 119 patients. Nearly all children in this series were treated with kilovoltage radiation. The high energy radiation of Cobalt[60] beams was used in just a few selected cases that were treated between 1955 and 1958. We now treat our brain tumors with megavoltage almost exclusively.

Our program of radiation therapy in children is almost the same as in adults, except that tumor doses administered in children are usually lower by a factor of approximately 20 per cent. Accordingly, average tumor doses of 4500 to 5000 rads in 45 to 50 days have been rarely exceeded in this age group. High energy radiation or megavoltage should be used. In children treated only by irradiation, this is ordinarily initiated as soon as the diagnosis has been established. When a child is first subjected to craniotomy and surgical removal of his tumor, irradiation is commenced approximately 2 weeks later.

RESULTS FOLLOWING IRRADIATION OF BRAIN TUMORS IN CHILDREN

Radiosensitivity

Primary brain tumors are all radiosensitive initially, more or less like most primary malignancies in children. The younger they are, the more radiosensitive. However, it must be noted that radiosensitivity is not synonymous with radiocurability. Immediate clinical improvement is usually observed early after the onset of treatment, an amelioration often dramatic. When a child's condition is critical because of increased intracranial pressure, decompression is urgent. Radiation therapy should be initiated immediately after decompression and must be considered an emergency procedure in some cases. Most children respond quickly and improve to such degree that by the time radiation therapy is completed, a full clinical recovery ordinarily can be observed.

Overall Survival and Recovery Rates

The assessment of treatment results in children with primary intracranial tumors rests upon the same 2 essential criteria that we have used consistently: length and quality of survival.

The length of survival has been estimated in all cases from the first day of radiation therapy. No correction has been made in survival or recovery rates on account of death by accident or unrelated diseases. Clinical follow-up is complete up to 1964 in all 119 children irradiated for their brain tumors more than 5 years ago (Table 11), and up to 20 years or longer (Chart 3).

Chart 3

PRIMARY   INTRACRANIAL   NEOPLASMS   IN   CHILDREN

LONG TERM SURVIVAL AND RECOVERY RATES SUBSEQUENT
TO ADEQUATE IRRADIATION USED POSTOPERATIVELY OR ALONE*

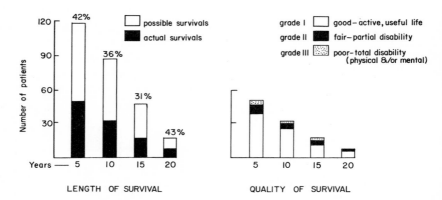

LENGTH OF SURVIVAL   QUALITY OF SURVIVAL

*From children adequately irradiated under 15 yrs. of age, 66% postoperatively, 1939-58: (follow-up complete)
to 1964

At the time of this report, the longest survival period among those that we have treated during infancy or childhood has attained 23 years from the time of irradiation. This patient was 5 years of age when irradiated post-operatively for a cerebellar astrocytoma incompletely removed. Presently, she is living and well, working as a qualified dietician. She is not alone in her class, as there are 5 more of our former children who are alive and well over 20 years after intensive irradiation for brain tumors.

The 5-year survival rates are shown (Table 11) for all children in accordance with the histologic category and the anatomic location of the primary brain tumors that we irradiated as part or all of their treatment. The percentages seen in that table make it quite obvious that the proportion of 5-year survivors in certain types of tumors is higher than in others to a degree probably unsuspected. It must be noted that no percentage is under 25 per cent, the lowest being in brain stem tumors which are reputed to have the worse prognosis, inasmuch as tumor location is concerned. In our overall series of 119 children, 50 have survived over 5 years, a grand percentage of 42 per cent (Table 11 and Chart 3).

Most significant are the following data from a detailed analysis of our survivals in children. It may be surprising to many that 42 of our 50 5-year survivors are still living as follow: 13 between 5 and 10 years from the onset of irradiation, 15 from 10 to 15 years, 8 between 15 and 20 years, and 6 over 20 years. Only 8 of the children who have survived over 5 years have deceased: 7 died of late tumor recurrence and one of unrelated disease. In 5 of the 7 5-year survivors who died of tumor recurrences, this happened between 5 and 7 years from the time of treatment, and in the other 2 children tumor recurrence was the cause of death nearly 10 years after onset of treatment.

A graphic presentation of the length and quality of survivals side by side is worthwhile studying (Chart 3). The rates are shown on a quinquennial basis at the end of 5, 10, 15 and 20 years after treatment. This is an overall assessment for all types of primary brain tumors exposed to adequate irradiation, either after or without surgical procedure, in children 15 years of age or under, from the time of their first radiation treatment.

Survival rates considered alone are gratifying. It is particularly so, in view of the fact (Table 11) that 74 of the 119 children treated over 5 years ago had tumors in categories recognized as rather unfavorable. Furthermore, patients were often in critical condition at the onset of radiation therapy. Among the 119 children irradiated for brain tumors over 5 years ago, 86 were treated for over 10 years, 45 over 15, and 14 over 20 years. Survival rates (Chart 3) indicate substantial long-term salvage rates.

Survival rates have more significance when evaluated together with the degree of recovery. Treatment results among infants and children, under the prevailing conditions, may be truly meaningful only when a substantial majority of long-term survivors have made a good recovery. These survivors must be able to live an active useful life. Very few have been living as destitutes, mentally or physically, or both.

Recovery rates have been re-assessed every 5 years among the survivors over 10, 15 and 20 years (Chart 3). An analysis of the quality of survival or degree of recovery among the children who have exceeded 5 years of survival has shown that 80 per cent of the 5-year survivors returned to normal and useful life and remained well through the years. Partial disability continued from the time of diagnosis and treatment in 16 per cent of the cases. Total disability, physical only, remained in approximately 6 per cent of the children, that is in only 3 of the 50 who have survived over 5 years. Of 86 treated for more than 10 years, 31 (36 per cent) have exceeded a 10-year survival and only one of 31 remained totally disabled and continued to be so until he expired over 15 years after treatment.

To the best of our information there is not a single florid mentally deficient as yet among the long-term survivors still living (42 of 50 5-year survivors) as detailed in a paragraph above. It would seem that our post-irradiation brain tumor patients, treated during infancy and childhood, have grown physically and developed mentally as well as any other group of comparable size might have done if picked at random in the general population.

From the standpoint of possible endocrine disturbances, which might be associated with indirect radiation effects on the pituitary gland, gross clinical evidence of such late radiation complications is rather scanty. There were 3 or perhaps 4 patients who may have had an earlier puberty than

usual, 1 boy and 3 girls. We are not aware of any late case of hypo-
gonadism or hypothyroidism in our series. We know of at least 6 children
among those who have become adults that are now married and raising a
family. One just had her fourth child, having been treated 19 years ago
with radiation alone for a proven medulloblastoma. It is estimated that
her pituitary gland must have received a tumor dose of approximately
3000 rads in 30 days, such dose being incident to the irradiation of her
tumor in the posterior cranial fossa.

Combined Surgical Removal and Irradiation

In children under 15 years of age, irradiation was administered postoperatively in 66 per cent of all our cases. Brain tumors irradiated postoperatively consisted of all the glioblastomas, unclassified gliomas, astrocytomas, ependymomas, the majority of medulloblastomas, and the
minority of mid-brain and brain stem tumors. Most of the few non-
gliomatous tumors were treated by combined surgical removal and postoperative irradiation.

One quarter (30 cases) of the primary brain tumors in the present series
consisted of gliomas of astrocytic origin (Table 11). The few glioblastomas responded poorly no matter where located. The intermediate group
of astrocytic tumors or unclassified gliomas have reacted favorably and
given a 5-year survival rate of 36 per cent for tumors within that group.

It is obvious (Table 11) that in children the highest 5-year survival rate,
75 per cent, occurred in the astrocytoma group of primary intracranial
tumors. But it must be kept in mind that 8 of the 12 5-year survivors in
that group are children who were irradiated postoperatively for cerebellar
astrocytomas and that surgery alone might have been sufficient to accomplish the same results. The remaining 4 patients with astrocytomas were
irradiated for cerebral hemispheral tumors of the non-cystic or diffuse type
that had been incompletely removed.

Favorable results were achieved in children with ependymomas: 5 of 7,
or 71 per cent, have survived over 5 years following treatment with
combined surgical removal and postoperative irradiation. There was no
oligodendroglioma in our series of children.

Regarding the management of the non-gliomatous tumors in children,
the incidence is low as these represent an average of 9 to 10 per cent of all
primary intracranial tumors in patients under 15 years of age. The histologic variety is limited. Non-gliomatous tumors in children consist mostly
of cerebellar sarcomas, craniopharyngiomas, and the odd pinealoma. Most
of those tumors are ordinarily treated by combined methods. The experience of others and ours has been presented in the previous chapter to
which I would like to refer the reader.

Treatment Principally by Irradiation Alone

Radiation alone was used to treat 41 or 35 per cent of our 119 children. Primary brain tumors treated only by irradiation consisted of the majority of brain stem and mid-brain tumors, plus 10 medulloblastomas and 2 cerebellar sarcomas.

In the treatment of mid-brain tumors in children we are depending, in our center, more and more upon the effects of adequate irradiation. Of 14 children, 9 were treated for tumors in that anatomic location by irradiation alone, all since 1952. Five of these 9 children have survived over 5 years, and 2 of these have already exceeded 10 years. Not one of the 9 children with mid-brain tumors was treated long ago enough to have attained 15 years of survival as yet. Three of the 5-year survivors have made a perfect recovery. The others are partially disabled. It seems that children with mid-brain tumors have had better results, so far, when treated by irradiation alone than with combined surgical removal plus irradiation. Of 5 children treated by surgery followed by irradiation, 3 have survived over 5 years and 1 of these 3 has surpassed the 10-, 15- and 20-year marks, being alive and well over 20 years after combined treatment.

Of 20 children with brain-stem tumors 18 were treated by irradiation alone. Of these 18, 3 have survived over 5 years and are still living in good condition over 8, 15, and 20 years respectively since treatment. Only 2 were treated by surgical extirpation and irradiation. These 2 were found to be astrocytomas. Both patients, who were 6 years of age at the time, have grown nicely since, being alive and well over 8 and 9 years from the time of treatment.

In view of the absence of natural anatomic separation between mid-brain and brain stem, tumors developing in children from these parts of the central nervous system could be combined together as we did above (Chart 2b) for all tumors in such location regardless of the method of treatment. Results show that 13 of 34 children or 38 per cent have survived over 5 years. Only 2 of these 13 have died. The remaining 11 5-year survivors are living, 6 of these between 5 and 10 years, 2 between 10 and 15 years, one over 15 and 2 over 20 years from the time of treatment.

Regarding medulloblastomas and sarcomas in children, these have been discussed at length in preceding Chapters 5 and 7. Intracranial sarcomas seem to be the only group of tumors which did poorly in comparison to the results observed in adults.

Of the 37 children treated by irradiation alone 12 or 33 per cent have survived over 5 years. All of these 12 children who have survived over 5 years up to 23 are still living: 6 between 5 and 10 years, 3 between 10 and 15 years, 2 between 15 and 20 and one over 20 years.

The degree of recovery has been remarkably good among those 12 children who survived more than 5 years after treatment by irradiation alone. None developed tumor recurrence as yet. Not one is mentally disabled or insane. All have grown normally from the somatic viewpoint. Only 2 have not recovered fully from the symptoms and neurologic deficit that they presented prior to irradiation, even though they have shown some improvement. Both have to move around in a wheelchair in which one is taken to school. They were treated 6 and 7 years ago by irradiation alone for mid-brain tumors, at the ages of 2 and 5 respectively.

Comparison of survival rates was made between the children treated only by irradiation and those treated for gliomas of the same categories with surgery followed by irradiation. The 2 groups were comparable in size, 37 and 34 children, and composed of the same types of tumors. The results of this comparison clearly reveal that survival rates between the two groups are identical at 5 years, but are appreciably higher at 10, 15 and 20 years among those who were treated solely by irradiation more than 10, 15 and 20 years ago. Our experience indicates that children who have been treated for medulloblastomas, mid-brain and brain stem tumors have survived longer and have attained long survivals in a higher proportion when actively treated solely by adequate irradiation.

CHART 4

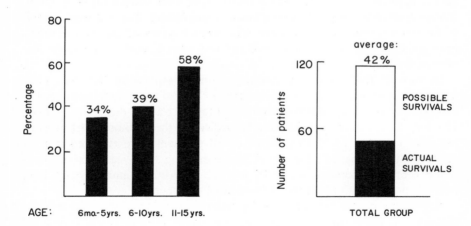

5 YEAR SURVIVALS

Primary Intracranial Tumors Irradiated in Children Under 15 Years of Age

Influence of Age Factor at Time of Treatment

We were curious to try to find out whether there might be any difference in 5-year survival rates in relation to the age of infants and children at the time they were irradiated for their brain tumors. This analysis suggests that in gliomas, regardless of the treatment used, the older a child was the higher the survival rates and the better the prognosis (Chart 4). The favorable difference in 5-year survival rates appears to be particularly significant in the group of children who were treated between the ages of 11 to 15.

COMPARISON OF RESULTS BETWEEN ADULTS AND CHILDREN

In a previous report[15], our experience in regards to children irradiated in the treatment of brain tumors was first presented. It was then stated that, in general, children can be expected to do as well and probably better than adults in terms of longevity and useful survival. Further analysis of this comparative study has just been completed, by considering separately and side by side the long-term survival and recovery rates in adults and in children. This was done after introducing an additional 5-year group of patients treated for more than 5 years and followed completely like all the previous cases in our series. The impression that we had gained at the time of that previous report is definitely confirmed at this time (Chart 5) now

CHART 5

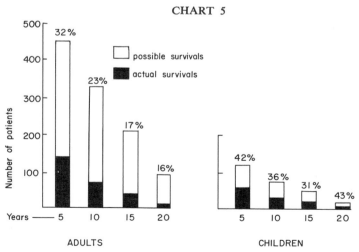

Total of 564 adequately irradiated pts. in 1939–58 ---- 119 (21.1%) were children under 15 years of age at the onset of irradiation

Irradiation of Primary Intracranial Neoplasms—Comparison of Postradiation Survival Rates in Adults and Children

that we have more cases available for review and longer periods of observation in the follow-up of our patients. We believe that the number of cases studied is large enough to be statistically significant. A close scrutiny of the difference in results between adults and children suggests that several factors may be accounting for it. One of these factors is the difference in incidence of glioblastomas which is low in children and high in adults, so that the latter group has sustained heavy losses from these highly malignant tumors. Another factor which has contributed to a higher salvage rate in our group of children seems to be directly related to the increasingly better results that were achieved in the management of medulloblastomas as well as mid-brain and pontine tumors, in which losses of life can be so heavy in children. There can be no doubt in our minds that such reversal in the prognosis of children affected with brain tumors, still considered hopeless by many, is mainly attributable to adequate irradiation in the management of their tumors.

Autopsies of Children Who Died Subsequent to Treatment of Brain Tumors

Autopsies were performed in 18 or 26 per cent of 69 children who have died. These happened to be performed at different periods of time following irradiation ranging from a few months to over 10 years. Postirradiation brain necrosis which had been suspected clinically was confirmed by autopsy in 1 patient. (see case report, p. 38).

In conclusion, our survival and recovery rates in children affected with malignant intracranial neoplasms have demonstrated beyond any doubt that such neoplasms can be irradiated adequately without fear of undue sequelae. In children, no appreciable disturbance of normal growth and mental development resulting from therapeutic irradiation of the brain and brain stem has been observed in 119 children included in the present analysis of results. One child died from brain necrosis following retreatment for tumor recurrence 5 years after initial treatment. Although in the majority of these children the pituitary gland could not be protected and has probably received as much radiation as the primary neoplasm itself, there is no detectable evidence that this important gland has been adversely affected in any of the 50 children who have been followed for at least 5 to 20 years and over from the time of irradiation.

To achieve adequate irradiation with virtually no postirradiation complications in children, it is our firm conviction that increased intracranial pressure must be controlled with effectiveness. Furthermore we believe that irradiation must be accomplished in a single protracted course with an optimum dose-time-volume relationship.

The present series illustrates well that the beneficial effects of radiation therapy in children treated for brain tumors can be considerably greater than their rare potential adverse effects.

9

Radiation Therapy of
Metastatic Intracranial Tumors

THE INCIDENCE of brain metastases represents 1 to 5 per cent of all cases of cancer, according to Chao, Philips and Nickson[18]. It appears that the incidence of intracranial metastases is increasing steadily, although it remains rare in children. A series of 389 cases was reported by Richards and McKissock[96], and their cases formed a group of 10 per cent of all verified intracranial neoplasms seen at their institutions during 1946 to 1960.

Primary Sites of Malignant Growths
Metastasizing to Brain Most Frequently

The primary sites of malignancies metastasizing intracranially most frequently are changing from time to time, and perhaps from one part of the world to another. In countries where bronchogenic carcinoma is detected with an increasing frequency, metastases to the brain may be identified more often than ever before. In certain parts of Asia, primary nasopharyngeal carcinomas occur frequently. Yet, blood borne cerebral metastases rarely ever occur from carcinomas so close to the brain, even though these currently invade the base of the skull through which they permeate into the cranial cavity and occasionally the brain itself by direct extension. Ho[44] has examined and treated some 3000 patients with nasopharyngeal carcinomas and stated that he has never seen a proven case of blood borne brain metastasis.

The sites of origin of carcinomas which send metastases to the intracranial parts of the central nervous system vary considerably. Carcinomas involving certain organs metastasize intracranially more often than others. Actually there is a constant predominance of cerebral metastases originating from the lungs and bronchi, followed by those from breast and kidney. Elvidge and Baldwin[32], in an analysis of 88 consecutive neurosurgical cases of metastatic tumors involving the central nervous system, found the

167

primary sites of growth in that order of frequency. Since their report, the incidence of bronchogenic carcinoma has continued to rise in many countries and this was bound to reflect on the frequency of brain metastases. Störtebecker[109] reported on 158 patients with brain metastases of which 30 arose from hypernephromas.

Richards and McKissock[96], in the analysis of their 389 patients with secondary intracranial tumors collected from 1946 to 1960, found that 252 cases or 65 per cent of their series originated from bronchogenic carcinoma. Diagnosis of the primary site was made during life by biopsy in 190 and at necropsy in the 62 remaining cases of cerebral metastases originating from carcinoma of the bronchus. It is notable that in 17 per cent no primary tumor was detectable on the radiographic examination made on admission. The primary sites of the other metastasizing growths were identified as follow: breast in 23 patients or 6 per cent, gastrointestinal tract in 19 or 5 per cent, and kidney in 11 or 3 per cent. Primary tumor sites responsible for intracranial metastases remained unknown in 66 cases or approximately 17 per cent.

DIAGNOSIS OF CEREBRAL METASTASES

Presumptive or Confirmed Diagnosis

The diagnosis of brain metastases is often made on a clinical basis only, upon the knowledge of an identified or else a probable primary malignant tumor unknown as yet. Evidence of an expanding intracranial lesion may be the first and sole manifestation of a primary carcinoma whose site was unsuspected until a brain metastasis was discovered. In such cases, the intracranial metastatic implant may be undistinguishable from a primary brain tumor. Symptoms and signs may suggest a single focus of intracranial disturbance. They may be somewhat incongruous, lacking in coordination and point to multiple foci of disturbance at once. Symptomatology is therefore variable, inconsistent and asystematic. The duration of symptoms may be quite different from one case to another depending upon the primary site of the metastasizing growth. Richards and McKissock give an average of 3 months' duration for symptoms of brain metastases due to bronchogenic carcinoma, and 4½ months for carcinoma of the breast. Elvidge and Baldwin[32] have expressed the opinion that, from the clinical point of view, the predominant location of metastatic deposits was the cerebral hemisphere in carcinoma of the lung or bronchus, and also of the breast.

The histologic diagnosis of brain metastases may be determined during life or at necropsy, or else never confirmed. In the series of 252 verified intracranial metastases from carcinoma of the bronchus that Richards and

McKissock[96] reported, histologic verification was obtained during life in 190 patients of whom 78 moreover were examined at autopsy. In 62 cases, the presumptive diagnosis of cerebral metastases was verified at necropsy only.

Biopsy of intracranial metastases may be associated with a high mortality and morbidity. Of 123 patients subjected to biopsy only, Richards and McKissock have reported that 84 or 68.5 per cent of those with brain metastases from carcinoma of bronchus, breast, kidney or uncertain origin lived one month or less.

Solitary or Multiple Intracranial Metastases

When a cerebral metastasis is suspected, it is essential to try to determine whether the lesion may be solitary or associated with other intracranial tumor implants.

The incidence of solitary brain metastases from bronchogenic carcinoma was found by Galuzzi and Payne[38] to be 13.9 per cent of 741 autopsies on patients who died of that primary malignancy. Among 61 necropsies on patients who died of a bronchogenic carcinoma and in which Richards and McKissock disclosed evidence of intracranial metastases only, 24 solitary and 37 multiple tumors were found.

From 59 necropsies on patients with intracranial metastases originating from other sites than the bronchus and the lung, 9 solitary metastases were found, an incidence of 15.2 per cent (Richards and McKissock). That incidence rate is only slightly higher than the 13.9 per cent found by Galuzzi and Payne[38] in their large series of necropsies on patients who died of bronchogenic carcinoma. Those and other series are in accord that solitary brain metastases from various types of carcinomas may be expected in approximately 15 to 20 per cent of all cases of brain metastases.

The incidence of single intracranial metastases may be lower and the prognosis more severe when other visceral metastases are associated with single intracranial tumors. In an overall group of 147 necropsies made on patients who died of bronchogenic carcinoma, 39 or 26.5 per cent had solitary brain metastases. Among 86 cases in which other visceral metastases were associated, single intracranial metastases were less frequent and found in 15 cases or 17.4 per cent (Richards and McKissock).

Advantages and Limitations of Special Examinations

Various investigative procedures may be helpful in demonstrating the presence, location and perhaps multiplicity of brain metastases. Special examinations, however, have definite limitations, as generally they cannot

PLATE 8

Outline of the head showing contour brain scan pattern in a series of parasagittal concentric arcs (technique of Feindel, Yamamoto, McRae and Zanelli [34]).

Inverted "V"s indicate left sided local differential uptake of Risa at level of metastatic choriocarcinoma in the central temporoparietal area.

On (a) scan before combined therapy with metrotrexate and radiation (Cobalt[60]).

On (b) scan after treatment showing non-significant diffuse uptake suggesting tumor disappearance.

PLATE 8

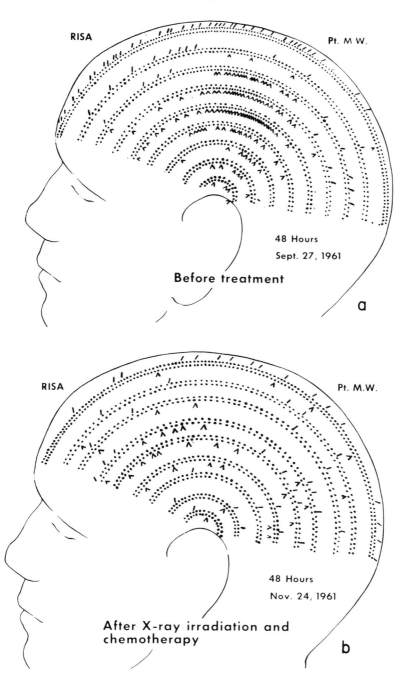

RISA

Pt. M W.

48 Hours
Sept. 27, 1961

Before treatment

a

RISA

Pt. M.W.

48 Hours
Nov. 24, 1961

After X-ray irradiation and
chemotherapy

b

PLATE 9

a and *b*, Brain scan showing differential isotope uptake in right cerebellar region, representing a solitary lesion proven to be a metastasis from carcinoma of the breast.

H.B., a 73-year-old lady was admitted to the M.N.I. 4 years after right radical mastectomy for adenocarcinoma. Three months prior to admission she developed occipital headaches, nausea, vomiting and ataxia. Left carotid angiogram was within normal limits. Pneumoencephalogram revealed moderate hydrocephalus. Ventriculography showed expanding lesion in the right cerebellar hemisphere. Metastatic adenocarcinoma was found at operation.

c and *d*, Brain scan illustrating uptake of Mercury 197 by 3 separate lesions, one in the right cerebral hemisphere, and two in the left. At operation all three proved to be metastatic melanomas. Other metastatic nodules were found in the left parietal region but were too small to be picked up by the scanner.

R.M., 43-year-old male, was admitted to the M.N.I. 5 years after removal of small melanoma from right inframmammary region. Right parietal headache and left lower visual field defect. On right carotid angiogram, a medium sized expanding lesion was found in the right parietal lobe. Left carotid angiogram was negative.

Four weeks later he was readmitted with right hemiparesis and dysphagia. Brain scan made on second admission revealed at least three focal spot uptakes at that time.

e and *f*, Scan demonstrating differential isotope uptake in both cerebral hemispheres. At autopsy the lesions were found to be metastatic nodules from bronchogenic adenocarcinoma.

F.D., 52-year-old male, was found to have in the right posterior chest a mass causing pain in the area. At thoracotomy, the right lung was removed and the mass proved to be a primary circinoma. His condition deteriorated rapidly. A search for brain metastasis disclosed the presence of two metastatic lesions in the right posterior temporal and the left occipital regions. Diagnosis was confirmed at autopsy.

PLATE 9

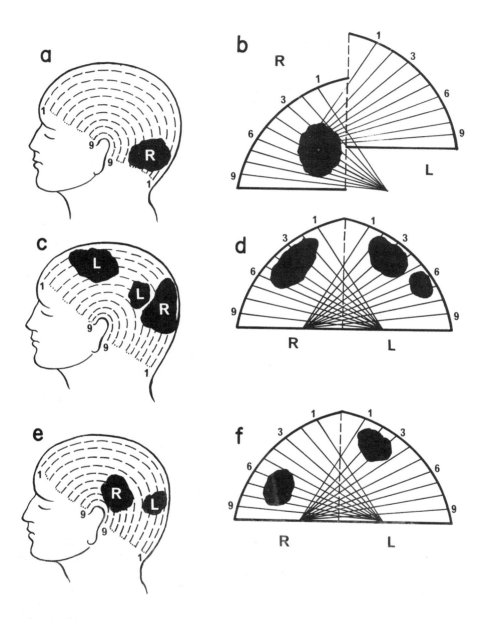

assist much in determining the nature of a solitary lesion, whether primary or secondary. Those diagnostic techniques can, but infrequently, establish the existence of more than one lesion when brain metastases are suspected. This is usually true of air studies. Angiography may be useful in demonstrating a network of fine neoformed capillaries which may be visualized either in glioblastomas or in metastatic tumors. When this is found on angiograms in only one region of the brain, it does not allow differentiation between the two types of tumors. If a similar pattern were visualized in more than one area, such finding would practically be diagnostic of multiple metastases. Electroencephalograms are often useful in showing evidence of multiple foci of disturbance of brain activity in the presence of multiple metastatic deposits.

Gamma encephalogram is probably the most useful method of investigation of suspected intracranial metastases. Radioisotope brain scans are capable of demonstrating multiple metastatic cerebral implants more often than any other method. The main limitation is the size of the metastatic nodules which must exceed 1.5 to 2 cm. to be demonstrable (Plates 8 and 9). Gamma encephalograms may reveal the distribution of metastatic deposits in one or both cerebral hemispheres and at times lesions located in the posterior fossa.

The presence of demonstrable visceral metastases other than intracranial must be known in determining the overall clinical picture before reaching a treatment decision. Chest films and radiographic skeletal surveys are necessary. Radioisotope liver scan should also be included.

Brain Metastases Simulating Primary Neoplasms

Metastatic tumors may infiltrate the brain in a way such as to simulate a primary tumor at operation. This has occurred in cases of single expanding intracranial lesions before a primary carcinoma could be suspected, even less discovered. Such instances happened not only in the gross examination of tumors but were confirmed by microscopic examination of the histopathologic sections as well. That illustrates to what extent the diagnosis of brain metastases may be difficult at times.

Ten cases of cerebral metastases simulated primary intracranial tumors so completely that these lesions were histologically diagnosed and subsequently irradiated as primary tumors of various histological types (Bouchard and Peirce)[15]. It happened in tumors rather diffuse and anaplastic in character. The histologic diagnoses available at the time of initiation of treatment consisted of the following classes of primary brain neoplasms: 2 glioblastomas, 2 astrocytomas, 1 undifferentiated glioma, 1 ependymoma, and 1 medulloblastoma among the gliomas, whereas the non-gliomatous tumors comprised 1 perithelial and 2 meningeal sarcomas. The original diagnoses were rectified subsequently. Review and comparison of the tissue sections revealed that the neoplastic lesions, previously treated by a combination of surgery and irradiation, were not primary brain tumors but metastases from carcinomas. The 10 cerebral metastases, which had simulated primary brain tumors, originated in carcinomas arising from the bronchus in 3, from unknown sites in 2, and from breast, thyroid, testis, ovary and rectum in the remaining cases.

Richards and McKissock[96] reported that 4 tumors thought to be gliomas from the biopsy histology were found at autopsy to be brain metastases.

The fact that a single expanding intracranial metastasis may occasionally simulate a primary neoplasm, not only clinically but histologically as well, should not be too surprising. The following case report illustrates how this can happen. A girl, 13 years of age, had a craniotomy for a cerebellar tumor which was removed as completely as possible. The histologic diagnosis was medulloblastoma. Postoperatively, her entire cranial and spinal contents were adequately irradiated. The girl made a good recovery and remained well for 3½ years. She was then readmitted to hospital for lumbar pain which was presumed to be due to tumor implant along the spinal axis. Clinical investigation revealed cervical lymphadenopathy and multiple bone metastases. An ovarian tumor was found, which was removed surgically and proved to be a dysgerminoma. Review of the histopathologic evidence demonstrated that the initial manifestation of this dysgerminoma had been an intracranial metastasis which histologically resembled a primary medulloblastoma.

INDICATIONS FOR TREATMENT AND RESULTS

The clinical management of cerebral metastases must be considered a palliative problem essentially. Relief or improvement of the mental and physical condition of patients affected with brain metastases is the prime objective. Prolongation of useful life following physical as well as mental recovery may be accomplished in most cases, but the duration of such improvement is unpredictable and may vary substantially. Dramatic results have been observed frequently. The selection of the method of treatment must be judicious.

Surgical Extirpation of Single Metastasis

In the management of intracranial metastases, surgical extirpation is indicated and should be attempted, if feasible, when the clinical evidence available suggests a single or solitary lesion located in a region from which the tumor could be extirpated. Surgical approach is particularly indicated when a single metastasis may originate from a primary malignancy which is well differentiated and usually considered radioresistant, for instance a melanosarcoma or perhaps an adenocarcinoma of the stomach. Such treatment decision is applicable when the identity of the source of the lesion may be suspected from a known history of carcinoma, or else when at the time of operation extemporaneous biopsy brings histological evidence.

A single intracranial neoplasm in a patient over 60 years of age may be a primary neoplasm, but is strongly suspicious of being a solitary metastasis until histologically verified at operation. Single metastatic lesions in the brain may represent approximately 15 to 20 per cent of all intracranial metastases. One must also be aware that even when clinical and other evidence is strongly suggesting a solitary brain metastasis, there is always the possibility that there may be multiple intracranial lesions particularly when other visceral metastases are present.

The fact that a metastatic lesion may be solitary does not mean that it can be extirpated in toto. This appears to be feasible when the metastasis is found to be sharply demarcated, being more or less surrounded by a halo of edematous brain of hyaline appearance. Total excision of cerebral metastases was performed by Richards and McKissock in 108 cases or nearly 28 per cent of the 389 patients included in their report on treatment of intracranial metastases[96]. The mortality rate for total excision of metastasis was 32.2 per cent. Following total excision, 18 lived more than 1 year.

It would appear that not less than one third of the patients with solitary intracranial metastasis have lesions which are rather infiltrative in character. Such lesion cannot be extirpated in toto but only partially. Partial excision was performed in 56 cases in the total series of Richards and McKissock, and only 2 survived over 1 year.

Of a total of 22 patients who survived over 1 year after surgical treatment of solitary metastasis, 10 had a metastasis from bronchogenic carcinoma and 6 from breast cancer. Four were survivors following total excision of metastatic carcinomas of unknown origin. Two other patients lived over 1 year: one following biopsy only, and the other after total excision of a cerebral metastasis followed by the later excision of a cerebellar metastasis.

Richards and McKissock believe from their experience that surgical excision of an apparently single or solitary intracranial metastasis is worthwhile. This may be the case particularly when the metastasis manifests itself some time after the primary has been removed from the breast or kidney. It is possible that such surgical excision may complete a cure.

Palliative Irradiation of Brain Metastases

Radiation therapy should be considered as palliative treatment in the management of intracranial metastases to relieve symptoms and neurologic signs and also attempt to restrain tumor growth. Palliative irradiation should be used only when there is a reasonable chance that metastatic lesions can be controlled, so that a patient may achieve a relatively useful recovery and survival period. Irradiation may be used alone or postoperatively.

Irradiation alone should be considered in cases of solitary intracranial lesions only when surgical exploration and tumor removal have been rejected for reasons such as the poor general condition of a patient or the presence of other visceral metastases, particularly when vital organs are involved. Treatment only by irradiation is also indicated in cerebral metastases when these are multiple or bilateral, or else located in critical areas such as the mid-brain and brain stem. Palliative radiation therapy must be used particularly when brain metastases are deemed radiosensitive.

Palliative postoperative irradiation is indicated when a solitary tumor could not be removed completely or in cases operated upon who were found at operation to have multiple metastases which could not be demonstrated prior to operation.

The most gratifying palliative result that we have observed in the treatment of brain metastases was in a lawyer who had an orchiectomy followed by irradiation. One year later he developed severe headaches and became comatose. At craniotomy, there was an extensive metastasis involving the left temporal lobe, extending posteriorly through the mid-brain into part of the cerebellum. Partial removal of the tumor was accomplished for decompression purposes. Histologically the tumor presented the picture of a seminoma. The postoperative course was stormy. He was accepted for irradiation while still comatose. Response to radiation therapy of the entire intracranial content was remarkable. He completed his treatment as an ambulatory patient. A depth dose of 4500 rads in 39 days was administered. Apparently the tumor regressed almost completely. This remission lasted 5 years. Further brain metastases then developed and he was irradiated again to a depth dose of 5200 rads in 37 days. A second complete remission lasted 19 full months after which time he presented evidence of generalized carcinomatosis. Altogether this man lived just short of 9 years after initiation of treatment. For 7 of the 9 years he was able to carry a large portion of a heavy legal practice, an active community life as well as enjoy his family.

Radiation therapy combined with systemic chemotherapeutic agents may be more effective in certain cases particularly when metastases are multiple not only in the brain but also elsewhere in the body.

Chao, Philips, and Nickson[18] reported observations on 38 patients treated for palliative purposes with X-radiation. Because of the prevalent incidence of multiple metastatic lesions, they have used opposing lateral fields encompassing the entire area. In order to avoid increasing and excessive intracranial pressure, small initial daily doses have been used. In their experience, clinical improvement became manifest after approximately 1000 rads in the first week or 10 days. When palliation only was desired, tumor doses of approximately 2000 r were delivered but ordinarily the total dose was carried up to 3000 r in the hope of preventing recurrence of neurological signs. Good palliative results were obtained in 63 per cent of the 38 patients treated.

We have reported in a previous publication[15] some of our observations after irradiation of 29 patients for metastatic lesions involving the brain or the brain stem. Since then, no further review of our clinical material was made in respect to brain metastases. Ten patients, in that series of 29, initially received radiation therapy as a postoperative procedure following clinical and histologic diagnosis of primary intracranial neoplasms of various types. These 10 cases subsequently proved to be metastases and have been discussed in a previous paragraph. Of the 19 remaining patients, 16 presented a known history of primary malignancies. Three patients were considered as having cerebral metastases and treated as such, despite the fact that no definite primary malignant tumor could be demonstrated. The histologic diagnosis was confirmed in 9 cases, 7 by craniotomy and 2 by needle biopsy. Treatment was administered on the basis of a clinical diagnosis in the remaining 10 patients.

The effects of radiation therapy in the management of brain metastases are generally worthwhile. The majority of patients, over 75 per cent, have experienced relief of symptoms early. Only 7 of our entire group showed no improvement at all. Ordinarily, clinical improvement manifests itself by relief of headache, gradual disappearance of neurologic signs and return to consciousness within 8 to 15 days from the onset of irradiation. Our clinical observations in that respect have been similar to those reported by Chao, Philips, and Nickson.

Patients recover physically and mentally and usually remain well for most of the duration of their survival. The longest survivals that we have observed lasted 102, 86 and 51 months from the onset of radiation therapy. Ten other patients survived over 1 year, whereas 16 lived less than 1 year. The degree of recovery was good during the major part of the survival of 17 patients, fair in 5 and poor in the 7 remaining.

Technique of Irradiation

In general, radiation therapy of intracranial metastases aims to control and restrain growth of multiple tumor implants. The entire intracranial content should be exposed to radiation in all cases. This has to be done because 80 to 85 per cent of brain metastases consist of multiple lesions of which only the larger ones may be demonstrable and cause symptoms or signs.

We rarely ever use doses under 2000 rads over a period of approximately 21 to 28 days, the dose being estimated in mid-line of the cranial cavity. In treating metastases from tumors of moderate radiosensitivity, carcinoma of the breast for instance, exposures of 3000 to 3500 rads over 35 to 40 days are currently used. Exceptionally, in dealing with more resistant tumors such as well-differentiated squamous cell carcinomas, adenocarcinomas of the gastrointestinal tract, hypernephromas and melanomas, we may administer tumor doses up to 5000 to 6000 rads in 50 to 60 days, providing that patients present no evidence of visceral metastases other than cerebral. Megavoltage should be utilized whenever available.

Chemotherapy

Chemotherapeutic agents may be employed with efficacy in some of the patients with brain metastases. Drugs known to have selective effects on cells and tissues of any particular type of primary malignancy should be utilized in the treatment of secondaries in the brain. The use of various anticancer drugs seems to be indicated against fast growing anaplastic intracranial metastases, particularly when these are multiple, whether unilateral or bilateral.

Infusion methods of drug administration might be preferred when metastases are demonstrable in the brain only, despite the probability of metastases elsewhere. Systemic chemotherapy is rather indicated in patients whose intracranial metastases merely represent one of the many manifestations of more or less generalized carcinomatosis.

The biologic effects of drugs on intracranial metastases might be enhanced, if radiation therapy is combined with chemotherapy. The timing and dosage of irradiation must be carefully planned in relation to the mode of administration and the selection of drug.

In conclusion, palliative treatment of intracranial metastases may be worthwhile, inasmuch as many patients may regain consciousness and be relieved of their symptoms and neurologic signs. Often they return to a state of mental and physical improvement such that they can enjoy a good survival, whatever the duration may be. Survival periods seem to be under 6 months in about one half of the cases. Survivals of 1 year or longer can be observed in 10 to 15 per cent or more. A few long survivals will occur from time to time.

Surgical treatment should be considered primarily in all cases presenting satisfactory evidence of a probable solitary metastasis which might be enucleable.

Palliative irradiation of the entire intracranial content may be indicated when patients are considered inoperable or total extirpation has proved unfeasible at operation, or else cerebral metastases are multiple. Suitable doses of radiation may be really worthwhile in terms of temporary recovery and prolonged survival in good or fair clinical condition for most of its duration.

Selective chemotherapy alone or combined with surgical or radiotherapeutic methods may contribute to better and longer palliation of patients with intracranial metastases.

10 Treatment of Tumors of the Pituitary Gland

RADIATION THERAPY, used alone or in combination with surgery, holds a paramount place in the control of tumors of the hypophysis. Once the tumor growth appears to be restrained, hormonal management prevails. The proper treatment of tumors of the pituitary gland depends largely upon the knowledge and experience of each consultant in a team of specialists which should group endocrinologists, neurologists, neurosurgeons and radiologists.

In the treatment of patients affected with pituitary tumors, the prime objective is the suppression of adverse pressure effects on the surrounding glandular components within the hypophysis itself, and on adjacent extrasellar structures such as the optic chiasm and the hypothalamus. This must be accomplished with the minimum hazard to the patient's life and the maximum probability of correcting, in full or in part, the physiopathological disturbances created by a given type of pituitary tumor. The consultant therapeutic radiologist must be knowledgeable in the physiopathology of the hypophysis. He must also be familiar with the biological effects that ionizing radiation may induce not only in the normal and abnormal hypophysis but also in the adjacent structures.

My experience in the use of ionizing radiation for the treatment of primary pituitary tumors consists of 151 cases. Of those, 111 were treated more than 5 years ago and followed for periods varying from 5 to over 20 years. These 111 cases comprise 59 chromophobe adenomas, 36 eosinophilic, 9 basophilic and 7 miscellaneous tumors. There is only one primary malignant carcinoma of the pituitary gland in the present material. A few metastatic tumors involving the pituitary were treated palliatively by irradiation, but these were not included in the present figures.

The incidence of primary pituitary tumors represents approximately 8 per cent of all intracranial neoplasms. Pituitary adenomas are seldom encountered in children and adolescents. Primary tumors of the pituitary

181

gland manifest themselves predominantly between 30 and 45 years of age.

CHROMOPHOBE ADENOMAS AND HYPOPITUITARISM

Changing Concepts About Endocrine Activity

Chromophobe adenomas form the largest group of pituitary tumors under scrutiny. The onset of chromophobe adenomas is insidious. Clinical diagnosis is not made usually until a chromophobe tumor has reached a size sufficient to cause pressure on the normal acidophil and basophil cells and induce physiopathologic disturbances resulting ordinarily in hypopituitarism.

Until recently, chromophobe cells were believed not to produce endocrine secretion. However, concepts are changing. Hyperpituitarism has been reported in the presence of chromophobe adenomas which were considered responsible for Cushing's syndrome. This syndrome has also been observed with other histologic varieties of non-basophilic pituitary tumors.

When a pituitary tumor extends outside the sella, it may press upon the optic chiasm and cause secondary hemianopsia demonstrable by both clinical examination and visual fields. Visual complaints are the presenting symptoms in chromophobe adenomas in 60 to 65 per cent of the cases, and headache is in approximately 40 to 50 per cent.

Hypopituitarism Caused by Other Expanding Lesions

Hypopituitarism is more frequently associated with a chromophobe adenoma of the pituitary gland than with any other intracranial lesion. It must be emphasized, however, that the same clinical syndromes may be induced by several types of intracranial lesions which may directly or indirectly cause pressure on the pituitary gland and depress its functions. Craniopharyngiomas, which are usually located above the sella turcica and may represent 2 to 2.5 per cent of all intracranial neoplasms, are probably the most common lesions simulating a chromophobe adenoma. Hypopituitarism can be induced also by the following intra- or extrasellar lesions: cysts arising in the gland itself or in the stalk, hypothalamic lesions, suprasellar meningiomas, optic chiasm gliomas, parasellar carotid aneurysm and chordomas growing from the basisphenoid.

Impairment of vision is more frequent with chromophobe adenomas than any other type of pituitary tumors. Radiographically, enlargement of the sella turcica is a common finding, the incidence being approximately 92 per cent. The enlargement has been described as ballooning in type with intrasellar tumors. Encroachment upon the sphenoid sinuses may be found

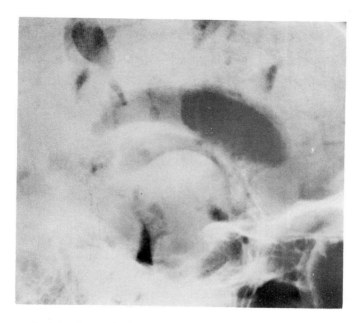

Figure 9, On lateral encephalogram, a proven chromophobe adenoma much larger than expected is clearly outlined with gas, the tumor bulging considerably above the sella, elevating the floor of the third ventricle and stretching the optic chiasm. This encephalogram illustrates the need for air studies prior to treatment decision, particularly before treating solely by irradiation.

in about 50 per cent of the cases. When disturbances of the visual fields are present, pneumoencephalography is extremely useful and nearly essential to determine the size and extent of a suprasellar tumor (Fig. 9). Arteriography may be required to assist in the differential diagnosis and exclude the presence of a carotid aneurysm when a parasellar lesion might be present (Fig. 10). Those methods of investigation often are of considerable assistance in arriving at a firm clinical diagnosis before selecting the appropriate method of treatment.

TREATMENT OF CHROMOPHOBE ADENOMAS

The treatment of chromophobe adenomas may consist primarily of either surgical removal solely or irradiation alone, or else a combination of both methods in which irradiation is commonly used postoperatively.

Surgical Removal Only

Treatment of chromophobe adenomas by surgical extirpation only is

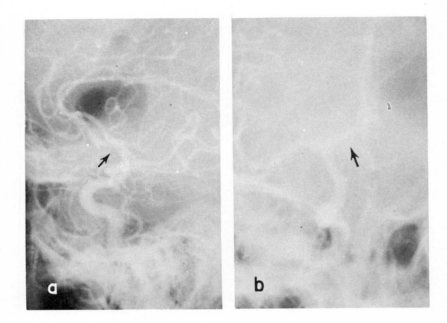

Figures 10 a and b, On lateral and antero-posterior carotid angiograms, displacement of the anterior cerebral artery by chromophobe adenoma. The size of the supra-sellar extension can be demonstrated more accurately from air studies.

capable of controlling some chromophobe adenomas. Horrax[46] reported on 54 patients who were operated upon without previous or subsequent irradiation. Twenty-eight or 52 per cent have lived from 5 to 20 years, and 23 of these 28 patients have remained well for the duration of their survival. In this series of Horrax[46] only chromophobe and chromophile adenomas were included in the report, but the proportion of chromophobe adenomas was not stated. Sheline, Boldrey and Phillips[105] have published their results in 95 previously untreated chromophobe adenomas. Among those, 34 patients were treated by operation alone. Of 17 patients who survived operation and improved postoperatively long enough to be available for follow-up observation, 11 had recurrences. In this series there are only 7 patients remaining under observation and currently without evidence of recurrence. In final analysis, only 4 of their patients treated by operation alone have remained under control for more than 5 years, whereas 3 were recurrence-free for less than 5 years at the time of their report.

Combined Surgical Removal and Irradiation

In studying Cushing's 338 cases of pituitary tumors, Henderson[43] stated that good results following frontal surgical procedure can be prolonged and some of the recurrences prevented by postoperative roentgen therapy. He showed that the 5-year control rate increased from 57.5 to 87.1 per cent with postoperative irradiation. Horrax[46] reported that 22 of 25 patients who were given a course of irradiation following surgical removal of their adenomas lived 5 to 16 years, and that 18 of them maintained their clinical improvement over the corresponding span of time. Sheline *et al.*[105] had 28 of 34 patients irradiated postoperatively for chromophobe adenomas which remained under control for periods of 5 years or longer, a 5-year remission rate of 83 per cent.

In our series of chromophobe adenomas treated more than 5 years ago, 28 patients had surgical extirpation of tumor combined with postoperative irradiation. Twenty-three have made a good recovery and remained free of recurrence (Table 12). Further analysis of our results has shown that 4 patients had little or no improvement following combined treatment and 3 of these survived less than 5 years. The fourth patient lived over 18 years, but over these years he was operated 3 times and irradiated as often. A fifth patient was well for 16 years before developing a recurrence for which he had a second operation; he is still alive and enjoying good health. The remaining 23 patients, or 82 per cent in this series of 28, have remained well and recurrence-free: 5 over 5 years, 10 over 10 years, 7 over 15 years, and one over 20 years (Table 12).

Treatment by Irradiation Alone

Radiation therapy alone has been used in the management of tumors diagnosed as chromophobe adenomas. There are several reports in the literature showing that chromophobe adenomas treated by irradiation alone may respond favorably and remain under control for long periods of time. The duration of periods of remission without recurrence is not always clearly defined. Objections to treatment by irradiation alone are mostly the selectivity of patients and the lack of histologic verification. It is recognized that other types of lesions than chromophobe adenomas may present analogous clinical pictures and that a careful differential diagnosis must be accomplished before treating patients solely with radiation.

Chromophobe adenomas treated by irradiation alone, in a single course of treatment with tumor doses of 3000 to 3600 roentgens in 25 to 30 days, were reported by Kerr[57]. Excellent or good results were achieved in 70 per cent of 37 cases followed for more than 5 years. Horrax[46] reported 88 per cent improvement or tumor control after tumor doses of 4000 rads in a series of 66 patients, but the period of follow-up observation was short, being from 1 to 6 years. Correa and Lampe[23] obtained satisfactory results in 56 per cent or 36 of 64 patients treated by irradiation alone.

We have treated by irradiation alone 28 chromophobe adenomas available for review 5 years or longer after treatment. Analysis of our results indicates that 3 patients died without improvement, even though they survived over 2, 3, and 8 years respectively following irradiation. Five other patients had recurrences 6 to 12 months subsequent to radiation therapy.

The most significant finding in our analysis is that 20 patients treated by irradiation alone have never required any further treatment. They remained recurrence-free for 5 years or longer, a rate of 71 per cent. Of these 20 patients, 10 were irradiated between 5 and 10 years ago, 8 between 10 and 15 years, and 2 between 15 and 20 years (Table 12).

Management of Recurrences of Chromophobe Adenomas

When recurrences of chromophobe adenomas happen, they are usually within the first few and rarely over 3 to 5 years following treatment. Most of our own recurrences have been observed 6 to 12 months subsequent to radiation therapy. Sheline et al.[105] believed that few recurrences are to be expected among patients remaining under control for 5 years or longer. The higher the rate of control after irradiation, the more patients may be expected to enjoy long periods of recovery with persistent arrest of tumor growth. Among those irradiated postoperatively, we have observed only 2 patients with late recurrences 10 years or longer.

There appear to be 2 main factors responsible for recurrences of chromophobe adenomas: the incidence of cystic components within the tumor itself or the invasive character of some neoplasms. Cystic chromophobe adenomas have been reported to occur in 10 to 40 per cent of the cases. The average incidence is approximately 20 per cent. Henderson[43] reported that hemorrhagic cysts were more frequent than the xanthochromic types. Sheline et al. reported that cystic tumors were found at the initial operation in 24 of 80 patients; 9 were hemorrhagic and 15 non-hemorrhagic.

Some chromophobe adenomas are solid tumors which may grow to be large and aggressive in character. Such pituitary tumors are called "malignant chromophobe adenomas" because of their behavior. Histologically they are considered atypical, but are not true carcinomas. Malignant chromophobe adenomas usually extend through the capsule of the tumor and may invade the adjacent structures by direct infiltration of the cerebral lobes, the temporal in particular. This was actually the case in a patient mentioned above who was operated on 3 times and had postoperative irradiation just as often over a survival period of 18 years. Several authors have reported cases of malignant chromophobe adenomas.

Judging from our experience in the treatment of recurrent chromophobe adenomas, it appears that surgical management is primarily indicated, irrelevant of the initial mode of treatment. After treatment by surgical removal alone, 3 patients not included in our present series were irradiated when tumor recurred. Not one of these showed improvement even though they were subjected to very adequate doses of X-radiation.

Following combined treatment, we have indicated above that 4 patients had little or no improvement. One of the 4 lived over 18 years, but during those years he was operated 3 times and irradiated as often. A fifth patient developed late recurrence 16 years after initial combined treatment. He was then operated for the second time, and is still alive and enjoying good health.

Among patients treated by irradiation alone, we had 3 who died without improvement or further treatment. Of 5 patients who had recurrences subjected to surgical extirpation, complete remission of symptoms followed in all. None of the 5 patients ever showed signs of further reactivation of their chromophobe adenoma. Three of them are alive 10, 15, and 23 years from the time of initial treatment, whereas 2 survived 15 and 18 years before dying of unrelated disease. Of the entire group of 28 patients whom initially we had planned to treat solely by irradiation, the only one who has survived over 20 years as yet is one of those 5 patients who had postirradiation recurrence treated by surgical removal; this man is presently alive and well 23 years after initiation of treatment. It is our opinion that surgical treatment seems to be superior to irradiation in the treatment of recurrence of chromophobe adenomas when adequate irradiation has been used before, either alone or postoperatively.

EVALUATION OF TREATMENT RESULTS

Clinical Improvement and Arrest of Tumor Growth

The efficacy of treatment methods in the management of chromophobe adenomas should be estimated on the basis of the criteria suggested by Sosman[107]. The criteria were as follow: recovery of vision, restoration of health, return to normal mode of living, and duration of overall improvement.

The majority of patients suffering of headaches at the onset of irradiation were relieved during the course of treatment or in subsequent weeks.

Most patients with visual field defects began to experience improvement about the second or third week from the onset of radiation therapy. Our records show that treatment by irradiation had to be interrupted within 2 weeks of commencement in 2 patients only who were operated on to relieve pressure on the optic chiasm, because their vision was continuing to fail rapidly.

During a course of radiation therapy, it is not too unusual for a patient to present symptoms of considerable lassitude, general weakness and mental depression. Acute panhypopituitarism may be responsible for such clinical picture. This has occurred in not less than 3 of the older patients treated by irradiation alone, approximately 3 to 4 weeks after onset of treatment (when dose levels reached 2500 to 3000 rads). Such condition was remedied satisfactorily by the administration of corticosteroids.

The rates of recovery of visual field defects have been reported by several authors, sometimes with substantial variations. After operation alone, Sheline et al.[105] have observed visual field improvement in 68 per cent of their cases. Following combined surgical treatment and post operative irradiation, Richmond[98] has reported some form of visual improvement in 87 per cent of patients. Subsequent to irradiation alone the rate of improvement reported by Correa and Lampe[23] was 60 per cent, whereas Sheline et al. had 54 per cent.

Correction and improvement of endocrine depression or imbalance related to treatment of chromophobe adenomas continues to be difficult to determine by hormone tests and assays for many reasons. The lack of sensitivity of many of the tests is one of these, on account of the wide variations between normal and abnormal levels. Another reason stems from the fact that replacement hormone therapy continues to be required for the correction of hypopituitarism effects in most patients.

From the standpoint of gonadal depression, several males treated with radiation alone recovered libido and potency. Some female patients who had been amenorrheic for some time began to menstruate again without replacement hormonal therapy. At least one became pregnant and had normal pregnancy and offspring.

The restoration of the sella turcica must not be expected as an index of the efficacy of treatment of pituitary adenomas. Unger and Roswit[114] have recalled that recalcification of the sella is rather unusual. In reporting 3 exceptional cases of apparent repair of the sella, they reviewed the literature in that respect. Bachman and Harris[5] had pointed out that of 64 patients they had treated, not one enlarged sella was seen to have decreased in size. Demineralized clinoid processes have shown no radiographic evidence of recalcification.

Replacement Hormone Therapy Required

The clinical results of treatment of chromophobe adenomas may be determined by the degree of recovery gained by patients following the attempts made to relieve their symptoms and signs of endocrine disturbances in target glands. When the thyroid, adrenals, and gonads fail to resume their normal functions, replacement hormone therapy must be attended to by endocrinologists. The hormonal balance may or may not be reestablished, depending upon the degree of temporary or permanent perturbation induced by the tumor directly within the hypophysis itself, or indirectly on the target glands.

Pituitary tumor growth appears to have been arrested when the endocrine clinical situation has eventually become stable. A clear indication of efficacy of the treatment method applied to control the primary lesion responsibile for hypopituitarism may be expressed by the duration of survival. Far more significant is the duration of the period of recovery, without any further sign of reactivation. In other words, once patients have improved and the tumor growth is apparently arrested, the most important yardstick for the evaluation of treatment of chromophobe adenomas is the recurrence-free rate.

Survival Rates in Chromophobe Adenomas

Assessment of treatment results on the basis of survival rates is not considered a valid yardstick by many in the management of pituitary tumors. Many years ago, Sosman[107] pointed out that survival periods of 3, 5, and 10 years were no criterion to evaluate the results of radiation therapy in pituitary tumors.

Our long-term survival rates have been tabulated side by side for chromophobe and eosinophilic adenomas (Table 13). The rates shown at 5, 10, 15, and 20 years following treatment have revealed no great difference between the two types of pituitary adenomas. It seems obvious that high survival rates are not necessarily reflecting the efficacy of the methods of treatment, any more than they are true indices of the morbidity of pituitary tumors.

Survival rates show a sharp decline beyond the 20-year period after treatment. That should not be surprising in relation to normal life expectancy. Perhaps the decline is sharper and occurs earlier than among normal individuals, a question to be decided by statisticians.

Recurrence-Free Rates Over 5 to 20 Years Following Treatment

Recurrence-free rates are valid standards of comparison for the evaluation of methods of treatment. In most reports on chromophobe adenomas, recurrence rates following surgical treatment alone are high, even though few have exceeded 50 to 60 per cent. The incidence of recurrences and the speed with which these develop have been reduced considerably by combining postoperative irradiation with surgical treatment. The reports mentioned above, including our own, have shown recurrence rates varying from 12 to 18 per cent in chromophobe adenomas irradiated post-operatively.

Richmond[98] believes that surgery followed by adequate irradiation is the method of choice and that all chromophobe adenomas should be treated in that manner. His opinion is based upon 220 cases of pituitary tumors, a large proportion of which consisted of chromophobe adenomas. Correa and Lampe[23] are of the opinion that no significant difference exists

TABLE 12.   Pituitary Tumors
Patients Improved and Recurrence-Free

| Follow-up Over | Chromophobe (56 cases)* | | Eosinophilic (32 cases)** |
	Surgery and Irradiation (28 patients)	Irradiation alone (28 patients)	Irradiation alone (32 patients)
5 Years	5	10	8
10 "	10	8	6
15 "	7	2	5
20 "	1	0	7
Total Improved and Recurrence-free	23	20	26
Rate	82%	71%	81%

* Not included are 3 patients irradiated for treatment of tumor recurrence, several years after surgery only.
** Not included in this total are 4 patients treated by surgery plus irradiation, which controlled 3 of the 4.

in results obtained by surgical treatment plus irradiation or by radiotherapy alone.

Our own series (Table 12) reveals a higher proportion of patients who improved and remained recurrence-free for periods varying from 5 to 20 years or longer, among those treated by combined surgical removal and postoperative irradiation of tumor. The recurrence-free rates differ from 18 per cent to 29 per cent between postoperative irradiation and irradiation alone.

SELECTION OF TREATMENT METHOD

Morbidity Related to Method of Treatment

The morbidity associated with the use of any treatment method must be considered before reaching a decision. The treatment of chromophobe adenomas by irradiation alone can be achieved properly with virtually and practically no complications. Even though operative mortality from surgical extirpation for pituitary adenomas has reduced considerably in most centers, it is still in the vicinity of 3 to 5 per cent.

The selection as to which method of treatment should be used first, whether surgical extirpation or irradiation, must be made in each case of chromophobe adenoma. The size of a tumor and the degree of pressure that it may exert on the extrasellar structures particularly the optic chiasm and the floor of the third ventricle should be the decisive factors.

Surgical Extirpation First or Irradiation Alone

Surgical exploration and management should be considered first when suprasellar findings suggest the probability of a cystic lesion or a large solid tumor, so that the diagnosis of chromophobe adenoma remains doubtful, despite suitable investigation. This therapeutic approach will have the advantage of surgical verification of diagnosis at the same time as decompression is achieved. We share with many others the opinion that cystic lesions are ordinarily not controlled as well nor for so long with radiation therapy alone as they can be by surgical removal first and irradiation afterwards. When a patient is becoming blind rapidly, surgical treatment should be used primarily to relieve pressure and give the nerve tissue a chance to restore and to prevent, if possible, permanent atrophy of the optic nerves and chiasm. If a tumor appears to extend into the floor of the third ventricle or temporal lobes, surgical treatment should be preferred and used first, because of the probability that it be a "malignant chromophobe adenoma" which must be extirpated before being subjected to irradiation for prevention of recurrence.

When irradiation alone is selected for treatment, it is essential to repeat visual field examinations often enough to determine whether there is regression or progression of the visual field defects. Results of treatment with radiation have been said to be less favorable in chromophobe adenomas than in other pituitary adenomas. It may have been so, but that seems to have changed considerably in the last 15 years due to the use of higher doses of radiation at tumor level. The advent of high energy radiation has apparently given more confidence to many in regard to the therapeutic potential of adequate irradiation.

Once the probability of a lesion other than a chromophobe adenoma has been excluded and there is no significant evidence of extrasellar extension, radiation therapy should be used first. Surgery should then be withheld for future use in the event that irradiation alone should prove incapable of controlling permanently a pituitary adenoma. Pressure on the optic chiasm by minimal or moderate suprasellar extension may be relieved with considerable efficacy by radiation therapy alone in the majority of the cases.

TECHNIQUE OF IRRADIATION

Adequate Doses of Radiation

There are a number of reports clearly stating that there is a direct relation between the results obtained and the doses of radiation delivered to the pituitary. The doses used 20 years ago are considered inadequate by the majority of therapeutic radiologists. In the last 2 decades there has been a gradual increase in tumor doses. After Kerr[57] multiple courses of radiation treatment have been discontinued in favor of single courses.

Bachman and Harris[5] showed the correlation of tumor doses with response to treatment in 6 cases. Correa and Lampe as well as Sheline *et al.* have expressed identical viewpoints. We are in agreement with the opinions expressed by the above observers. Doses varying between 4000 and 4500 rads and at times 5000 rads over a period of 40 to 45 days have been used consistently since 1946 and and are used presently.

Adequate irradiation with proper tumor doses can be accomplished well with kilovoltage. Megavoltage, when available, is advantageous by providing better depth doses in relation to the relatively small fields used. This also has the advantage of avoiding permanent epilation. We treat all pituitary tumors with Cobalt[60] radiation beams at 50 or 80 cm. focus skin distance.

Technical Beam Direction

Regarding the technique of irradiation, the size and number of fields directing radiation beams to pituitary adenomas preferably should be determined for each patient. This can be decided from the estimated size of the tumor, as judged from the degree of enlargement of the sella turcica and of tumor extension above it. The majority of chromophobe adenomas are well encapsulated and measure approximately 2 or 3 cm. in diameter. Fields averaging 4 x 4 cm. should be adequate for the irradiation of such volumes of tissue. With fixed fields the entire course of treatment may be administered by two lateral opposing fields. Positioning films are very useful and should be used routinely to control beam direction through the tumor-bearing area. It is difficult to conceive why so many are using lateral fields measuring 6 x 8 cm. covering areas of 48 square cm. to aim at tumors averaging 3 cm. in diameter.

When appreciable suprasellar extension is clearly demonstrated by pneumoencephalography, fields 5 x 5 cm. in size rarely need to be exceeded (Fig. 9). In such cases, however, anterior and posterior fields are often used to crossfire the pituitary tumor in order to avoid missing possible extension in the anteroposterior direction. Many are using beam direction devices which are more or less involved.

Rotational techniques are employed by several. Personally I use these rarely for the irradiation of pituitary tumors. This is because a substantial volume of normal brain tissue is exposed unnecessarily to doses of radiation which are still relatively high, even though decreasing, at the periphery of the rotational field in relation to the central dose delivered. This may be visualized by superimposition of the isodose curves obtained when direct lateral opposing small fields are used by comparison with concentric isodose curves resulting from rotation of the radiation beam (Plate 10).

PLATE 10

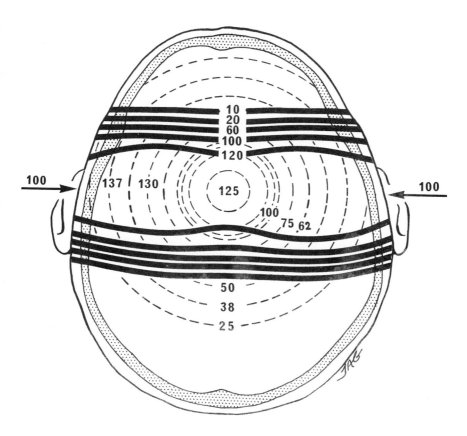

Irradiation of Pituitary Tumor—Superimposed Isodose Curves in Direct Lateral Opposing Fields, Compared with Concentric Curves in Rotational Technique

13

In summary, radiation therapy has become an essential part in the control of chromophobe adenomas. Doses must be adequate and should be administered in a single continuous course. Irradiation is indicated for the treatment of all cases. Long-term results have demonstrated that adequate irradiation alone can produce results nearly as good as when it is administered postoperatively. Surgical procedures should be used first and in all cases in which air studies have demonstrated appreciable suprasellar extension of any tumor arising from the sella turcica. Such lesions usually consist of large cystic or solid adenomas which will be dealt best by surgical decompression and extirpation. In all cases treated primarily by surgical procedures, postoperative irradiation is indicated.

EOSINOPHILIC ADENOMAS

Eosinophilic Hyperpituitarism and Acromegaly

Eosinophil or acidophil adenomas are small benign tumors developing in the anterior lobe of the pituitary gland. These adenomas are composed of proliferating eosinophil cells which are secreting growth hormone actively. Excessive secretion of growth hormone in adults causes acromegaly, a syndrome of eosinophilic hyperpituitarism. This abnormal production of growth hormone does not merely affect facial bones and extremities but viscera as well. Hypertrophy of the pancreas may be responsible for the high incidence of diabetes in acromegalic patients.

In acromegaly, moderate enlargement of the sella turcica is present in the majority of patients but may be absent in approximately 20 per cent. Eosinophilic adenomas may extend outside the sella turcica and press upon the optic chiasm and nerves in less than one half of the cases. For that reason, visual field changes are not a dominant feature of the acromegalic clinical picture.

Secondary Hypopituitarism

The increase in size of an eosinophilic adenoma is responsible for gradual mechanical pressure within the sella upon the rest of the glandular components of the hypophysis. This results in a depression of the other pituitary functions in relation to the target glands: thyroid, adrenals and gonads. Sooner or later signs of secondary hypopituitarism will begin insidiously to manifest themselves besides the evidence of eosinophilic hyperpituitarism which will continue to dominate the picture in the acromegalic patient.

CONSIDERATIONS ON TREATMENT

Therapeutic Objectives

The treatment of eosinophilic adenomas may vary in relation to the degree of functional activity of the tumor. The main therapeutic objective is the control of excessive growth hormone secretion by the adenoma. The second purpose is the relief of undue pressure by the adenoma within the sella, and beyond when required. Adequate control of secondary hypopituitarism and disturbances in carbohydrate metabolism must not be overlooked.

Some believe that conservative management and symptomatic treatment may be sufficient as long as the eosinophilic adenoma does not seem to be overactive and there are no pressure symptoms requiring immediate surgical decompression. Accurate determination of the degree of activity of an eosinophilic adenoma by its excess in growth hormone secretion has been most desirable. As yet, reliable growth hormone assays have not been readily available.

Selection of Treatment Method

Direct treatment of eosinophilic adenomas consists of irradiation alone mostly, and surgical removal plus irradiation. Surgical extirpation is usually incomplete, and inadequate when used alone. Selective total hypophysectomy in acromegaly has been successful in the hands of Ray and Horwith.[94]

Irradiation alone, when adequate, is capable of relieving symptoms and arresting tumor growth of eosinophilic adenomas in an increasing number of patients. This form of conservative treatment is currently applied with increasing efficacy. For many, the treatment of eosinophilic adenomas by adequate irradiation is now considered the treatment of choice. When tumors are bulky, surgical approach first is required to achieve decompression and remove part of the adenoma in most cases. Surgical treatment is usually combined with irradiation postoperatively.

RESULTS OF RADIATION THERAPY IN ACROMEGALY

Results of treatment in eosinophilic adenomas should not be assessed by the length of survival. Survivals of long duration are frequent (Table 13). This seems to be true even for untreated patients.

Control of Tumor and Growth Hormone Secretion

The main criterion of treatment efficacy is the evidence of arrest of tumor growth. Secretion in excess of growth hormone may then return to normal. Active signs of acromegaly should stop progressing, without, however, regressing.

Physical acromegalic signs are considered irreversible. Relief of headache may be expected in at least 80 per cent of the patients. Swelling of the soft tissues involving the face and hands may subside. Visual fields when affected will usually improve partially or even in toto. Those are the clinical signs of tumor regression and possible arrest of growth, but the salient external features of acromegaly persist. The unusual observation of a patient who had complete regression of acromegalic features and returned to normal status has been reported by Correa and Lampe.[23]

The apparent arrest of tumor growth following any treatment of an eosinophilic adenoma is not an infallible criterion of efficacy of the therapeutic method used. Periods of remission may occur spontaneously. Likewise, periods of discrete reactivation may intervene. These might be detectable by growth hormone assays and increase in serum phosphorus.

The incidence of diabetes is high in patients with acromegaly. Remissions after treatment may be interpreted as indirect indication that an eosinophilic adenoma is probably in a state of remission. In the management of acromegalic patients the control of diabetes is most important. Acromegalic patients do not seem to die directly from their pituitary tumors but they might indirectly from associated diabetes, hypertension, myocardial degeneration and renal failure.

Hormone replacement must be provided as required to correct the hormone imbalance induced by secondary hypopituitarism.

Recurrence-Free Patients After Radiation Therapy Alone

Results of treatment by irradiation were reported by Correa and Lampe[23] who have shown that these were good in 63.3 per cent of 31 patients with eosinophilic adenomas. In 11 patients, results were counted as poor. Seven survived over 10 to 15 years. They believe that no statistically significant difference could be demonstrated between results in the chromophobe and the eosinophilic patients. In their opinion, good results following radiation therapy have increased significantly with higher doses, ranging from 2000 to 2500 r up to 4000 r. When delivering large doses, 4000 r in 28 to 32 days, they like to use the high energy radiation of Cesium[137] or Cobalt[60].

In our experience with the treatment of eosinophilic adenomas by irradiation alone, 32 patients have been treated more than 5 years ago and followed completely. Long-term survival rates (Table 13) are amazingly high. Analysis of our results shows that tumor growth has been apparently

TABLE 13. Radiation Therapy in Pituitary Adenomas
Long-Term Survivals

Survival Over	Chromophobe			Eosinophilic		
	No. of Patients	No. of Survivors	Per Cent	No. of Patients	No. of Survivors	Per Cent
5 Years	59	53	90	36	32	89
10 "	41	32	80	28	20	71
15 "	19	15	79	20	13	65
20 "	11	4	36	9	4	44

arrested in 26 of the 32 acromegalic patients. Among these 26 patients, clinical improvement of symptoms has been observed without any subsequent detectable evidence of tumor recurrence or reactivation. Therefore, there was no need for any further treatment for tumor control, and this improvement persisted for the full duration of their survival. The rate of patients who have improved and remained recurrence-free indefinitely over 5 years after treatment up to over 20 years is 81 per cent in our series (Table 12). There are only 4 patients who were treated by surgery and subsequent irradiation in our experience with eosinophilic adenomas. Of the 4 patients, 3 improved and had no recurrence for the duration of their survival thereafter.

Management of Uncontrolled or Recurrent Eosinophilic Adenomas

Some patients with acromegaly fail to improve following treatment, whether by irradiation alone or combined surgical and radiological procedures. Others benefit of temporary remission of symptoms, without significant objective evidence of lasting arrest of tumor growth and control of hypersecretion of growth hormone.

In our series of 32 acromegalic patients treated by irradiation alone, we failed completely to control the disaese in 6. Severe headaches in the occipito-cervical or retro-orbital regions was the main complaint of each of the 6 patients who showed no improvement. Of these, 5 were subjected to craniotomy for relief of intrasellar pressure and extirpation of their pituitary adenomas. The splitting of diaphragms sellae, which were barely opened enough to allow passage for the pituitary stalk, seemed to relieve the intrasellar tension in 3 patients whose intractable headaches subsided. Extirpation of their eosinophilic adenomas at the same time seemed to control further active acromegaly. Intractable headaches persisted in the other 2 patients despite decompression of the sella and tumor removal, whereas clinical evidence of active acromegaly subsided in one but continued in the other.

One of the 4 patients treated surgically first and irradiated afterwards failed to improve, but received no other active treatment. The latter was found at autopsy to have a large pituitary tumor, mixed in type, invading the brain like some of the "malignant chromophobe adenomas" do.

Ray and Horwith[94] have subjected to total hypophysectomy 18 patients, 11 of whom had experienced only a temporary amelioration or else had not improved following x-ray therapy. The authors of that article reported no operative mortality nor major neurological complication. Of all the clinical manifestations, headaches were relieved dramatically, a result that they related to the effect of emptying the sella. The intracranial approach was used. The longest follow-up period was 7 years at the time of publication. So far they had good to excellent results in 15 patients who could be followed adequately.

Heavy Particles in the Treatment of Acromegaly

The work of Lawrence and Associates[66] in the therapy of pituitary tumors using the alpha particle beam from the synchrocyclotron at the University of California should be cited. They have felt that the heavy particle beam, as a source of external radiation therapy, gave definite advantages of greater depth dose deliverable to the pituitary gland with less scattering and more accurate delineation.

Since 1958, Lawrence et al.[66] have reported on 35 patients with acromegaly so treated. They used dosages ranging from 3000 to 10000 rads administered in 11 to 21 days. The present dosage used is 7500 rads in 12 days. Approximately 80 per cent of these patients were reported to have shown improvement in acromegaly both clinically and by target end organ hormone assays.

Lawrence et al.[66] have reported interesting changes in the carbohydrate metabolism following the treatment of those acromegalic patients. The results of standard glucose tolerance and insulin tolerance tests showed reversal to normal, 2 years or more after treatment, in 94 and 86 per cent of the patients who had abnormal tests when examined prior to heavy particle therapy. They have also found that circulating growth hormone levels were within the normal range following therapeutic applications of such particles to the hypophysis. This was verified in a group of 19 patients. They have also remarked that replacement hormone therapy was required in only 3 of 35 patients.

Technique of Irradiation

We have lived through a period of considerable evolution in the radiologic treatment of pituitary tumors. During the first 5 years of our series, we steadily increased our tumor doses to 3000 up to 3500 r, delivered in approximately 35 days. Nearly all our patients were treated in a single course, since only 5 received their treatment in repeated courses of lower doses. Presently we treat acromegalic patients with tumor doses of about 4500 to 5000 rads over 40 to 50 days, using megavoltage radiation (Cobalt [60]).

Irrelevant of the method of treatment used to control and arrest acromegaly, it must be borne in mind that secondary hypopituitarism is seldom corrected by the treatment applied primarily. Therefore it is important to prescribe replacement hormone therapy as may be required. As indicated above, other associated conditions, such as diabetes, hyperthyroidism and hypertension must be investigated and treated.

In summary, radiation therapy administered in adequate doses is capable of arresting the growth of eosinophilic adenomas and perhaps controlling excessive secretion of growth hormone. Such results should occur in approximately 80 per cent of the patients, for periods varying from 5 to 20 years and over.

Approximately 20 per cent of the cases were either uncontrolled or else recurred following irradiation. Such cases have been handled by surgical intrasellar decompression and extirpation of the pituitary tumor. Recent publication by Ray and Horwith[94] shows that total surgical hypophysectomy by the intracranial approach can be accomplished successfully. They achieved excellent results in controlling postradiation recurrences by trading apituitarism for hyperpituitarism of the type associated with secretion of growth hormone.

BASOPHILIC ADENOMAS

Basophilic Hyperpituitarism—Cushing's Syndrome

Pituitary adenomas consisting of basophil cells are not frequent. Because of their reported small size, basophilic adenomas may be present without causing appreciable enlargement of the sella turcica, but this seems to be true in only a certain proportion of the cases. Judging from our small series, enlargement of the sella might occur in 40 to 50 per cent of the patients. Baso-acidophil cells secrete a hormone known as adrenocorticotropic hormone or ACTH. In basophilic adenomas, secretion in excess of this hormone causes a syndrome described by Cushing as one of basophil hyperpituitarism, also called pituitary basophilism.

Secondary Basophilism—Cushing's Disease

The clinical picture of a patient with Cushing's syndrome is well known and quite characteristic. However, a disturbing factor results from the fact that an identical clinical picture may be present in a patient without a basophil pituitary adenoma. When this occurs, it is ordinarily in relation to adrenal tumors causing hypertrophy or hyperplasia of the basophilic cells in the pituitary gland with hypersecretion of ACTH. This physiopathologic process is then called Cushing's disease. According to Rovit and Berry,[101] the majority of patients presenting this syndrome spontaneously have bilateral adrenal hyperplasia. They also estimate that 15 to 20 per cent have adrenal tumors secreting ACTH causing their Cushing's syndrome.

Treatment of Basophilic Adenomas by Irradiation

Sosman,[108] in 1949, presented an excellent article on Cushing's disease and pituitary basophilism. He then discussed the role of radiation therapy and its beneficial effects in 4 of 6 cases. He clearly demonstrated that this syndrome may be reversible and can be controlled completely by external irradiation of the pituitary gland even though this does not occur in all cases.

Dohan, Raventos, Boucot and Rose[28] discussed the treatment of Cushing's syndrome, without adrenal cortical tumor, in a series of 12 cases in which they administered X-radiation to the pituitary region. Of the 12 patients, 5 had complete remission. In some, the signs of remission were mostly evident within 3 months. When there was no improvement, this could be determined within 6 months following treatment. Response was unsatisfactory in 7 of their cases, although 3 of these patients had partial remission of their clinical signs. Correa and Lampe[23] reported good response to irradiation in 6 patients with Cushing's syndrome.

External radiation therapy with heavy particles has been used by Lawrence and associates[66] in the treatment of pituitary tumors producing Cushing's syndrome. These workers have treated 5 patients between May, 1959, to 1965. The treatment conditions were apparently similar to those used in the treatment of acromegaly and mentioned above. They succeeded in suppressing the hyper-functioning of ACTH producing cells without restraining completely the production of the other trophic hormones. Clinical and endocrinologic improvement were observed. Menses usually return within 1 to 3 months following treatment. Patients require no hormone replacement therapy.

Internal interstitial irradiation of the pituitary gland has been achieved by Talairach and associates[112] in an attempt to control Cushing's syndrome. Using a stereotaxic method, they have inserted Yttrium[90] beads or seeds into the pituitary adenoma through the trans-sphenoidal approach. Between 1957 and 1961 they have treated 7 patients in an attempt to restrain hypersecretion of ACTH. Doses of 5000 to 10000 rads have been delivered to reach that objective. There was no operative mortality. Clinical and biologic results have been worthwhile. Four of their patients are enjoying a normal life without any additional or replacement therapy.

Author's Experience

In our series, 9 patients were treated with external radiation and followed for 5 years or longer. Clinical remission has been observed in 5 of them. The 4 remaining patients did not improve and died of complications associated with their syndrome. The first 3 patients that we treated had 1 or 2 courses of moderate doses of radiation directed to the pituitary gland. Total tumor doses were estimated to vary between 2000 and 3000 r over periods of 30 to 35 days.

We now treat in a single course, using Cobalt[60] radiation and tumor doses averaging 4000 to 5000 rads in 40 to 45 days. The last 3 patients so treated have now survived over 5 years in good condition without evidence of recurrence.

Altogether 6 of 9 patients have improved and 2 of them are living 15 and 20 years respectively after radiation therapy. The clinical picture may be fully reversible and some patients return to an apparently normal state of health without any other form of treatment. Females menstruate again. One of our patients became pregnant and gave birth to a normal child 18 months after irradiation for her Cushing's syndrome.

MISCELLANEOUS PITUITARY TUMORS, MIXED AND OTHERS

Mixed Adenomas and Hyperpituitarism

Mixed pituitary tumors are adenomas which histologically are composed ordinarily of both chromophobe and eosinophilic cells. Patients usually present variable degrees of hyperpituitarism due to increased secretion of growth hormone. They have the physical features of acromegaly combined with evidence of hypopituitarism. The exact diagnosis of mixed tumor is made at operation. This is how the diagnosis was established in 6 of the 7 patients comprised in our series. The other case was found to be a mixed pituitary tumor at autopsy. All our patients were therefore treated with external radiation postoperatively except for the latter who was treated solely by irradiation. Of those 7 patients, 5 have enjoyed long and good survivals varying from 7 to 15 years. The other 2 died 3 and 48 months following onset of treatment.

Mixed tumors consisting of chromophobe and basophil cells have been reported. A clinical picture of Cushing's syndrome is then seen as result of hyperpituitarism due to hypersecretion of ACTH. To my knowledge there is no mixed tumor of this type among our cases. Neither have we had any mixed adenoma in which the entire combination eosinophil-chromophobe-basophil was histologically demonstrated.

The clinical management of mixed adenomas should be identical to that of the dominant syndrome presented by the patient. We should aim to control hypersecretion of either eosinophilic or basophilic cells and induce tumor growth restraint and arrest. Suitable control of secondary hypopituitarism or other pathologic conditions must be attended.

Histologically Malignant Pituitary Tumors

Malignant primary carcinomas of the pituitary gland are rare. A recent follow-up study of Cushing's series of pituitary adenomas, published by German and Flannigan[40], shows that among 394 verified tumors there were 15 carcinomas, an incidence of about 4 per cent. Richmond[98] has reported 7 carcinomas in a total of 220 patients who received postoperative radiotherapy. He indicated a 5-year survival rate of 57 per cent in pituitary carcinomas treated by surgical removal followed by irradiation.

There is one proven case of adenocarcinoma in our series. Diagnosis was made at operation. Following partial surgical removal, a tumor dose of 6500 rads was given over a period of 68 days. Somewhat to our surprise this patient is alive and well 8 years after treatment.

Pituitary carcinomas must be kept separate from "malignant pituitary tumors." The latter, whether chromophobe, eosinophil, basophil, or mixed cell tumors are considered malignant not because of their microscopic histologic characters but on account of their invasive behavior and the difficulties encountered in controlling them, irrelevant of the method of treatment.

Metastatic tumors occasionally involve the hypophysis or develop in the sellar region. These may be suspected clinically but are more often found at autopsy. We have treated by irradiation a few cases diagnosed clinically and histologically proven later at autopsy. These were mostly in patients with metastases from carcinoma of the breast involving the base of the skull and cranial nerves, particularly the sixth. Diabetes insipidus occurred in at least 2 patients. Good palliative effect was achieved with external radiation directed to the corresponding area, using lateral opposing fields and depth doses averaging 2500 rads in approximately 4 weeks.

Although the following is not a case of metastatic manifestation, it might be interesting to mention a patient whom we have irradiated successfully for a number of lesions proven to be eosinophilic granulomas. More than 6 months ago, this 6-year-old boy developed diabetes insipidus which was attributed to another lesion of the same kind. Following irradiation of the pituitary region to a dose of 1500 rads over 12 days, this boy has improved markedly and remained under nearly complete control so far.

Cushing's Syndrome and Non-basophilic Pituitary Adenomas

The occurrence of Cushing's syndrome with pituitary tumors other than basophilic adenomas has been reported from time to time. Rovit and Berry[101] added to the medical literature 5 cases of Cushing's syndrome associated with proven non-basophilic pituitary tumors. At the same time, having gathered from the literature another 50 similar cases, they presented a study based upon a total of 55 cases. After discussing Cushing's syndrome in relation to basophilic and non-basophilic pituitary tumors, Rovit and Berry[101] have proposed a re-evaluation of pituitary tumors and hyperadrenalism.

Collation of the 55 cases of Cushing's syndrome associated with non-basophilic adenomas of the pituitary gland that Rovit and Berry[101] have reviewed and analyzed has revealed the following data. Of the 55 cases, 39 were considered as benign pituitary adenomas. Chromophobe adenomas have accounted for 29 of the benign types. Among the remaining 26 cases, they found 7 mixed adenomas, 3 "non-granular" and 13 "malignant" (predominantly chromophobe) pituitary adenomas; there were 3 adrenal cortical carcinomas associated with pituitary adenomas. Bilateral adrenal hyperplasia was found in 45 cases. Visual symptoms occurred in 31 or 56 per cent of the patients. Radiographic examinations showed an enlarged sella turcica in 55 per cent of 44 patients who had skull radiographs available. Hyperpigmentation of the skin was observed in 40 per cent of patients with Cushing's syndrome. This was considered related to excessive secretion of ACTH or MSH by the pituitary gland. Another interesting observation is that 10 of 39 patients who had benign pituitary adenomas developed hyperpigmentation following adrenalectomy. In respect to hyperpigmentation subsequent to adrenalectomy, the following case may bring some interesting clinical observations.

Case Report: Mrs. S.B., 34 years of age, was seen in consultation with a history of bilateral adrenalectomy for Cushing's syndrome due to adrenal hyperplasia. Following adrenalectomy she was placed on suitable medication. Seven years later, in July, 1962, she was complaining of blurring of vision, headaches, weakness and low abdominal pain of 2 weeks' duration. She reported that her skin had become dark. This was becoming more obvious with each menstrual period.

On physical examination, the skin was definitely hyperpigmented, a phenomenon affecting accessible mucosas as well. She was definitely obese. On roentgenograms of the skull, the dorsum sellae was eroded and the tuberculum undercut. The spine appeared demineralized in the thoracic and lumbar areas, and a compression fracture was demonstrated in one lumbar vertebra. The consulting endocrinologist made a diagnosis of melanodermia, presumably associated with hyperplasia of ACTH secreting cells in a chromophobe adenoma of the pituitary. It was agreed to treat this patient with external radiation.

Over a period of 53 days, she received a total pituitary dose estimated at 4750 rads, by crossfiring with four fields measuring 4 x 4 cm. in size, using megavoltage radiation (Cobalt [60]). The patient improved clinically. Hyperpigmentation of skin and mucosa has subsided appreciably in the 4 to 6 months following irradiation of the pituitary. At present time, more than 3 years after radiation therapy, she is well and symptom-free, but her melanodermia has not regressed completely as yet.

Following adrenalectomy, hyperpigmentation of the skin and increase in growth of pituitary adenomas with exacerbation of ACTH secretion have been known to occur. Rovit and Berry[101] reported that removal of a pituitary tumor in such cases was followed by a dramatic lightening of the skin in 7 of 11 patients, and this within a few months of the surgical extirpation of a pituitary adenoma. Postoperative irradiation of the pituitary region was accomplished in some cases. The authors have insisted that, in patients with "malignant pituitary tumors", therapeutic benefits were transient, irrelevant of the method of treatment.

The particular interest presented by the case just reported above lies in the fact that clinical remission of more than 3 years' duration has followed treatment, solely by irradiation, of a pituitary tumor presumed to be a chromophobe adenoma associated with Cushing's syndrome. From the point of view of radiation therapy, our patient was irradiated in the same manner as we ordinarily treat similar pituitary adenomas. It would be advisable, prior to irradiation, to determine by pneumoencephalography the size and the degree of extension of pituitary tumors when there are visual symptoms or else suspicion that the adenoma might be "malignant."

Galactorrhea and Pituitary Adenomas

The incidence of hypersecretion of lactogenic hormone or prolactin outside of normal periods of lactation does not occur frequently. Galactorrhea has been defined as any milk-like secretion which may occur, either spontaneously or else after pressure on the nipples, in non-puerperal clinical condition. Such milk secretion is usually a sign of endocrine disturbance, particularly along the pituitary-ovarian-mammary glandular interconnections. Other miscellaneous causes have been mentioned.

Bercovici and Eherfeld[9] have reported on 71 patients with non-puerperal galactorrhea. In 25 cases there were hypothalamic disorders. These were associated with a pituitary adenoma in 11 cases. Three other patients had acromegaly and one had a craniopharyngioma. Thus an enlarged sella turcica was found in 15 cases suggesting that galactorrhea may be an indication pointing to pituitary tumors. This syndrome can occur without a pituitary tumor. The fact that no appreciable sign of enlargement of the sella turcica and no other sign of a pituitary tumor can be found does not exclude the presence of small pituitary adenomas. Prolactin secretion may be attributed to eosinophilic cells in the pituitary gland; nevertheless eosinophilic adenomata causing acromegaly have seldom been accompanied by galactorrhea. Chromophobe adenomas are the types of tumors most frequently found when pituitary adenomas have been demonstrated in relation to galactorrhea.

Bercovici and Eherfeld[9] have not elaborated on treatment of galactorrhea. They have merely mentioned that some patients were given x-ray treatment. The following case report offers interesting observations in relation to irradiation of the pituitary gland in attempting to control intractable galactorrhea of long duration.

Case Report: Mrs. D. R., age 31, was seen for the first time in our department in June, 1964. Among her multiple complaints was persistent galactorrhea from the age of 18. She had first menstruated at 14, but subsequently her periods were irregular and scanty. About the same time she became overweight. At the age of 22, a diagnosis of Forbes-Albright syndrome was made and she was treated with estrogens. Her galactorrhea decreased but never stopped.

In June, 1964, she was admitted to the Department of Psychiatry for paranoid schizophrenia, suspected to be in relation with endocrine abnormality. Physical investigation was essentially negative. Assay for F.S.H. determination was negative at 6 m.u., a titer in keeping with a Forbes-Albright syndrome. After multiple consultations, endocrinologists concluded that her galactorrhea was part of a Forbes-Albright syndrome, presumably associated with a pituitary tumor yet to be demonstrated.

It was then decided to treat her pituitary gland with radiation. Over a period of 42 days, an estimated depth dose of 4664 rads was delivered with two lateral opposing fields 3 x 3 cm., using megavoltage radiation (Cobalt [60]). No change in her condition was observed from the onset of treatment in August, 1964, to the end of the year. Early in January, 1965, she reported that for the first time in 14 years her profuse galactorrhea had discontinued. When last seen she had had no further galactorrhea over a period of 15 months.

The physiopathology of non-puerperal galactorrhea remains at this time in the realm of speculation. In most cases, however, this disorder appears to be related to some degree of imbalance in the function of various endocrine glands. The excessive and untimely release of prolactin from normal or abnormal sources, such as pituitary tumors or other suprasellar influences, would seem to play an important part. In the above case it was presumed that a pituitary tumor yet to be demonstrated, probably a chromophobe adenoma, might be responsible for galactorrhea. An interesting response to adequate irradiation has been observed.

Irradiation of Pituitary Gland for Control of Remote Pathologic Conditions

Radiation Hypophysectomy in Generalized Carcinomas

In the palliation of advanced cancer of the breast, Lawrence and associates[66] have attempted to induce radiation hypophysectomy in 169 patients. High energy heavy particles were used. They have reported remissions ranging from 6 months to over 5 years, in about 30 per cent of their cases.

Radiation hypophysectomy has also been accomplished by internal irradiation within the sella turcica. Talairach *et al.*[112] have induced ablation of the pituitary by insertion of Yttrium[90] beads into the pituitary itself, aiming at its necrosis with doses of approximately 100,000 rads. They reported their results in 145 patients with osseous and visceral metastases from cancer of the breast. Satisfactory subjective and objective palliative effects have been accomplished. This method has also been used in the palliative management of prostatic carcinoma.

Diabetic Retinopathy and Radiation Hypophysectomy

Regression of diabetic retinopathy has been reported following surgical suppression of the pituitary gland. Several series of surgical hypophysectomies have been reported.

Many reports are available on radiation hypophysectomy achieved by intrasellar irradiation of the pituitary gland. The current method consists of insertion of Yttrium[90] seeds directly into the sella turcica using mostly the trans-sphenoidal route Talairach and associates[112] have reported some interesting results in that respect.

In the treatment of diabetic retinopathy, Lawrence and associates[66] have also used the 900 Mev alpha particle beam to destroy the hypophysis. They have treated in that manner over 100 patients. At present they use dosage of 12,500 rads in 12 days in attempt to suppress all pituitary function. Stabilization or improvement of retinopathy has been reported in 49 or 55 per cent of their 89 patients.

Malignant Exophthalmos and Pituitary Irradiation

The pituitary gland is considered capable of secreting an exophthalmos producing substance designated as E.P.S. Such substance, however, has not been isolated as yet.

Irradiation of the pituitary has been advocated and used in attempting to control malignant exophthalmos. Jones[48], in discussing the usefulness of orbital x-ray therapy in the management of progressive exophthalmos, reviewed the entire subject. He concluded that irradiation of the pituitary gland alone was ineffective after delivering doses of 1000 r in 11 days, the dose being estimated at level of the hypophysis itself.

Interstitial irradiation of the pituitary gland has been used by Talairach and his group in 4 cases of malignant exophthalmos. They have used doses of 5000 to 10,000 rads, using Yttrium[90] beads and Gold[198] seeds. Their aim was to depress the pituitary function and indirectly induce a regression of exophthalmos. It would seem that they have observed encouraging results.

Role of Radiation Therapy in the Management of Spinal Cord Tumors and Other Lesions

Incidence and Anatomic Factors in Cord Tumors

THE VALUE OF RADIATION therapy in the management of tumors and other lesions involving the spinal cord is difficult to determine. There must be very few observers who have irradiated and followed more than 50 patients with primary intramedullary gliomata.

The incidence of primary spinal cord gliomas in relation to all gliomas of the central nervous system is in a ratio of 1 to 15 according to Slooff, Kernohan and MacCarty.[104] Their study comprises 301 primary intramedullary tumors which represent 22.8 per cent of all primary neoplasms arising in the spinal canal.

The majority of primary neoplasms growing in the spinal canal, approximately 75 to 80 per cent, originate intradurally but develop outside the medulla itself. These extramedullary tumors are of mesenchymal origin and obviously occur far more frequently than primary intramedullary gliomas.

Metastatic lesions from distant malignant tumors are rarely found within the dural part of the spinal canal whether at operation or necropsy. In other words, intramedullary or extramedullary intradural metastases are seldom seen.

In the management of neoplastic diseases, extradural metastases are not infrequent. Through the intervertebral foramina, these invade and infiltrate the spaces between the dura mater and the rigid vertebral canal, affecting the cord indirectly by mechanical pressure.

A brief mention will be made of the role of radiation therapy in the treatment of syringomyelia and arachnoiditis.

RADIATION TOLERANCE OF THE NORMAL SPINAL CORD

Tolerance to Radiation of the Normal Cord

The question or radiation tolerance of the normal spinal cord came very much to the fore in 1948 following an article published by Boden[11] on radiation myelitis of the cervical spinal cord. For the first time, attention was focused on this potential complication. In a non-equivocal manner, with 10 well-documented and proven cases of radiation myelitis, Boden[11] demonstrated that it was not safe to unduly expose to radiation the normal spinal cord, and that such exposure occurred currently in the treatment of neoplasms of the head and neck. Radiation tolerance curves applicable to the brain stem and the rest of the human brain were published by Boden for the first time. The doses of radiation which, from Boden's curves, cannot be exceeded without risking radiation myelitis and cord necrosis have been mentioned in a previous chapter (see page 44).

Recently, Vaeth[115] has reviewed and discussed the problem of radiation-induced myelitis. He classified reactions of the irradiated spinal cord in three levels of severity. The first level of reaction is a transient myelitis, reversible in character, resulting from apparently mild radiation damage which may occur 1 to 12 months after irradiation, manifest itself over approximately the same length of time, and then subside. The second level is one of progressive myelitis, which becomes irreversible once established. Vaeth recalled the symptoms and neurologic signs. He insisted that radiation-induced myelitis should be differentiated from other lesions like metastases. The third and most serious level of myelitis is of such a degree of severity that it should never occur in the clinical practice of radiation therapy. In cases of progressive or irreversible radiation-induced myelitis, patients eventually die of complications resulting of treatment for a cancer which often has disappeared and may probably be cured. He concluded his study on radiation-induced myelitis by stating that "extension of treatment time appears to contribute the most towards preservation of normal tissues undergoing irradiation".

Reduced Radiation Tolerance of Cord Affected by Tumor

When treating tumors involving the spinal cord, particularly primary intramedullary gliomas, we are dealing with a diseased cord. The blood supply to the cord is already impaired to some degree, so that tolerance to radiation should be definitely lower than that of a normal cord. The radiation tolerance of a spinal cord involved with tumor growth must be expected to be lower than the safe limits indicated in any tolerance curve. Therapeutic radiation doses administered to the cord tumor must then be adequate without being excessive in relation to time and volume, lest pre-existing cord damage be aggravated by irradiation. Careful appraisal of the volume of tissue to be irradiated must be made in each case. A diseased cord is a highly vulnerable organ, being a small longitudinal structure with limited blood vessel circulation within itself.

Natural Cord Necrosis by Transecting Tumor

It must be realized that a primary spinal cord tumor is capable alone of causing necrosis of the cord in non-irradiated cases. Untreated gliomas of the spinal cord have been known eventually to cause transection of the organ and complete paraplegia. This is the natural behavior of untreated or uncontrolled spinal cord tumors.

In the management of 30 primary intramedullary histologically proven tumors of the spinal cord, we are not aware of a single case in which radiation transverse myelitis has occurred subsequent to postoperative irradiation. Since functional transection of the cord naturally occurs as result of damage caused by the neoplasm alone, and considering that many patients are paraplegic at the onset of irradiation, it would be practically impossible to differentiate between natural occurrence and damage partly due to super-added radiation therapy. In our own cases, irradiation might have played a part in the late evolution to complete paraplegia observed in 7 patients. This might have happened in the 7 patients who improved but remained partially disabled following surgical treatment combined with irradiation and became completely paraplegic after 3 to 7 years of partial improvement. This delayed paraplegia might just as well be attributed to tumor reactivation.

PRIMARY INTRAMEDULLARY NEOPLASMS

The Mayo Clinic Group Experience

Apparently, the first large series of primary intramedullary tumors of the spinal cord was reported by Kernohan, Woltman and Adson[54] when they studied 51 cases with an attempt at histologic classification. Later, Rasmussen, Kernohan and Adson[92] reviewed and classified 557 intra-spinal neoplasms, of which 11.5 per cent or 64 cases were primary intra-medullary tumors. Neurofibromas and meningiomas predominated, with a total of 303 cases. Their 64 cases of intramedullary tumors included 33 ependymomas and ependymoblastomas together with 10 astrocytomas. In a subsequent report presented by Woltman, Kernohan, Adson and Craig[119], 979 intra-spinal neoplasms were classified, from which there were 220 intramedullary gliomas or 22.5 per cent of the cases.

Slooff, Kernohan and MacCarty[104] have pursued the work of their predecessors and associates. Tumors of the spinal canal seen at the Mayo Clinic and histologically verified represent a total of 1322 cases. Of these, 29 per cent were neurilemmomas and 25.5 per cent consisted of meningiomas. Slooff et al. have concentrated their efforts on the review and study of primary intramedullary tumors of the cord and filum terminale. Their series comprises 301 cases, including 269 classed as primary gliomas and 29 non-gliomatous neoplasms. A brief review of this excellent work should prove to be highly informative and perhaps incite the reader to consult the original report.

The intramedullary gliomas reviewed by Slooff *et al.* comprise 169 cases classed as ependymomas, 86 astrocytomas, 8 oligodendrogliomas and a few mixed gliomas.

Intramedullary Astrocytomas. Nearly all these astrocytomas arise from the cord proper, as only 6 from a total of 86 were found in the filum terminale. Histologically, the majority, 76.7 per cent, were considered low in malignancy, being in Grade 1 (52.3 per cent) and Grade 2 (24.4 per cent). Only 5 cases appeared highly malignant and were classed in Grade 4. Pain was the presenting symptom in 68 per cent of the patients. Pre-operative duration of symptoms averaged 39 months in Grade 1 and 7 months in Grade 4 cases.

The treatment of intramedullary astrocytomas was surgical primarily, consisting of long laminectomy to relieve obstruction. Biopsy only was accomplished in 9 patients and total removal alone in 4, among 63 patients available for survival analysis. In the opinion of Slooff *et al.* the possibility of removing an astrocytoma of the cord is less than that of extirpating an ependymoma. Postoperative radiation therapy seems to be beneficial. Survivals, after operation, average 101 months in Grade 1 patients and shorten down to 12 months in the Grade 4. In dealing with primary intramedullary astrocytomas, comparison of treatment results based upon survival length in relationship to the extent of surgical treatment, with or without postoperative irradiation, is confusing and inconclusive.

Intramedullary Ependymomas. These spinal cord tumors form a group of 169 cases in the series of primary gliomas of the cord that Slooff *et al.*[104] have recently analyzed. Of the 169 cases, 108 were classed as histological Grade 1, whereas 36 were classed as Grade 2. Nearly 50 per cent of all ependymomas involved the filum terminale. The rest of them arose from the cord proper. The preoperative duration of symptoms averaged 56 months in the Grade 1 patients, and 33 months among those in the Grade 2 category.

At the Mayo Clinic, the surgical treatment of intramedullary ependymomas has consisted of laminectomy with longitudinal myelotomy between the posterior columns in order to expose neoplasms. Frequently, the surgeons were able to remove most of an ependymoma from the cord. Slooff *et al.*[104] have stated that postoperative irradiation seems beneficial. Survivals after operation averaged 151 months among the Grade 1 patients, and 101 months for those classed as Grade 2. Biopsy only was performed in 7 patients. Total removal was the sole treatment in 3 Grade 2 patients.

Postoperative irradiation was administered to 29 of 55 patients with ependymomas affecting the cord itself, and to 36 of 83 with ependymal cell tumors arising from the filum terminale. Slooff *et al.* have studied survival time of 138 patients in relation to the extent and nature of therapy. They have cautioned the reader that "interpretation of the data must be done carefully in that respect".

Other Data on Spinal Cord Tumors. The other histological types found in the series of primary intramedullary tumors reported by Slooff *et al.*[104] were small in number, consisting of 8 oligodendrogliomas and 3 mixed gliomas. The non-gliomatous tumors amounted to 10 per cent of all the primary intramedullary neoplasms. They have mentioned that they have found no primary spinal cord sarcoma in the literature and reported 1 case of fibrosarcoma arising from the filum terminale.

Primary gliomas of the spinal cord rarely metastasize to meninges. Unless a tumor continues to grow upward to invade the brain stem, its effect is to transect the cord. It has been suggested that the degree of malignancy cannot be estimated nor expressed in terms of postoperative survival. For several reasons, the value of roentgen therapy could not be assessed from their material.

Experience at the Neurological Institute of New York

Wood, Berne and Taveras[121] reported their experience with radiation therapy of intrinsic tumors of the spinal cord. In a series of 62 cases available for analysis, they had 39 pathologically classified tumors of which two thirds were ependymomas, and less than one third or 12 cases were astrocytomas. There were 4 miscellaneous verified tumors. The remaining 23 patients had surgical exploration so that their tumors were grossly verified; however, since no biopsy was taken, these tumors remained histologically unclassified. All unclassified tumors were intramedullary lesions. The authors felt reasonably certain that no case of syringomyelia was included.

Each of the 62 patients of Wood *et al.* were treated with radiation therapy during the immediate postoperative period. The time-dose relationship in the treatment of intrinsic spinal cord tumors was such that the median tumor dose per course was of 1700 r in 2 weeks. Repeated series of irradiation were given several months or years after the original course.

The authors recalled that the evolution of untreated spinal cord tumors is progressive, resulting eventually in crippling disability and death. The average life expectancy of patients treated solely by surgical procedures was estimated at 6 years by Wood *et al.,* on the basis of the Mayo Clinic series reported by Woltman and associates in 1951. In that respect, postoperative radiation therapy was considered beneficial to patients when these had shown evidence of clinical improvement with arrest of tumor growth, and had survived beyond the 6-year average length of survival just mentioned.

Of 23 patients irradiated postoperatively for ependymomas of the spinal cord, Wood *et al.* had 16 available for assessment, and 12 of these lived longer than the 6-year life expectancy of patients treated with surgical treatment alone, the longest survival being 19 years after operation. Altogether, 36 patients were suitable for assessment and 25 of them survived beyond the average 6-year life expectancy associated with surgical management alone. The grading for quality of survival showed that 43 of 58 lived in good, 8 in fair, and 7 in poor condition.

A Series From the Montreal Neurological Institute

Our experience with primary tumors of the spinal cord is based upon a series of 30 patients treated by irradiation postoperatively more than 5 years ago and followed completely up to 1964. In our series of primary tumors of the spinal cord, all cases were verified by surgical exploration and had either partial removal or biopsy. Histological diagnosis revealed the following types of tumors: 9 ependymomas, 6 astrocytomas, 8 unclassified gliomas, 1 glioblastoma, 3 meningeal tumors and 3 miscellaneous neoplasms (recurrent glioma of the filum terminale, fibrolipoma and teratoma).

Tumor distribution showed involvement of the cervical cord in 8 patients, thoracic in 16, and lumbar including filum terminale in the 6 remaining cases. More than one segment of the cord was involved at once in 2 patients. Not included is a recent case in which an intramedullary ependymoma was found that extended the length of the entire cord. This is suggesting a multicentric origin of the neoplastic process, which possibly developed simultaneously at every level of the cord ependymal canal.

Combined Surgical and Radiotherapeutic Procedures. Treatment of primary intramedullary tumors has consisted of surgical procedures initially. Laminectomy was performed to provide adequate decompression and exposure of the cord in every case. Some degree of surgical removal was achieved in 18 patients, whereas in the remaining 12 cases biopsy or cyst aspiration only were considered advisable.

Postoperative radiation therapy was administered in every case. The initial 5 patients in this series had short repeated courses of irradiation in the same fashion as the multiple course method described by Wood and his associates[121]. Subsequently, treatment by irradiation has been administered consistently in a single course with tumor doses equivalent to 4000 to 4500 rads over periods of 40 to 45 days, using kilovoltage radiation.

At present, megavoltage radiation (Cobalt[60]) is used in one continuous course, with tumor doses of approximately 5000 rads over periods of 45 days or longer but rarely exceeding 60 days. Such dosage is well within the

CHART 6

INTRAMEDULLARY SPINAL CORD TUMORS

LONG TERM SURVIVAL AND RECOVERY RATES ✱

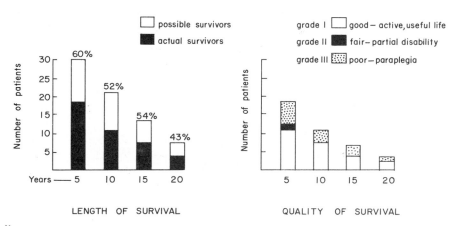

LENGTH OF SURVIVAL   QUALITY OF SURVIVAL

✱From 30 pts., verified surgically and histologically — all followed over 6 years

safe limits of radiation tolerance of central nervous tissue that can be extrapolated from Boden's curves. In view of the narrow width of the spinal canal, which seldom exceeds 3 cm., long narrow fields 3 or 4 cm. wide are considered suitable. Provision is made to include a good safety margin above and below the apparent extent of the intramedullary neoplasms to be exposed to radiation.

Survival and Recovery Rates Over More Than 5 to 20 Years. Analysis of immediate treatment results has revealed complete clinical improvement during the first year in 73 per cent of our patients, no improvement in 20 per cent, and partial improvement in the others. Of our 30 patients, 18 or 60 per cent have survived over 5 years. Not one of the 18 5-year survivors has lived less than 8 years from the onset of treatment, so that every long-term survivor in this group of ours has exceeded the average survival period of 6 years that Wood *et al.* have estimated for patients treated solely by surgical procedures for their primary cord tumors. Included among those 18 patients who have survived more than 8 years from the time of treatment, there are 4 who have lived over 10 years, 4 over 15, and 3 over 20 years (Chart 6).

The survival and recovery rates over 5, 10, 15, and 20 years are presented graphically, side by side, on Chart 6. Long-term clinical improvement has been more or less a matter of all or nothing, either with complete lasting recovery or else full paraplegia at once. An intermediate group improved at first and later developed paraplegia, between 3 to 7 years after operation and radiation therapy. Ten years after treatment, the degree of recovery has become definitive for each patient in that small group as shown on Chart 6. Beyond 10 years of survival, only 1 patient died of reactivation of spinal cord tumor.

All the 5-year survivors were followed for at least 8 years. Of the 18 patients who actually lived over 8 years after treatment, 13 are still alive. There are 9 of these 13 patients who are perfectly well: 2 over 20 years (the longest survival being 24 years since treatment), 4 over 15, and 3 over 10 years. Five long-term survivors died between 7 and 18 years, 2 of tumor recurrence and 3 of unrelated disease. Once a patient treated for a spinal cord tumor is a paraplegic, the quality of survival becomes a Grade 3. Yet, many of these patients may be relatively comfortable and can benefit by rehabilitation. The number of cases in the present series is not sufficient in each group to allow any statement as to which histological type may have obtained the best results over the years. Wood and his associates[121] have suggested that the prognosis for patients with primary intramedullary neoplasms was difficult to relate to the histology of the tumor.

In conclusion, it would seem that, in the management of primary intramedullary tumors, surgical decompression and exploration are indicated initially in all patients. Adequate postoperative irradiation is probably beneficial, contributing to arrest tumor progression and probably inducing regression as well. Combined surgical and adequate postoperative radiological treatment is apparently helping to restore normal function of the cord in an average of 50 to 60 per cent of the patients, largely on a lasting and perhaps permanent basis. All in all, this overall treatment management perhaps contributes to increase the average longevity of patients.

METASTATIC INTRADURAL TUMORS

Intradural metastases, either intramedullary or extramedullary, are rare findings. The diagnosis can be made solely by surgical exploration and biopsy. We have seen only 2 cases, one with metastases from cancer of the breast and the other with lymphosarcoma. The treatment should consist of radiation therapy directed to the spinal cord in the same way as in the case of primary cord tumor.

EXTRADURAL TUMORS

Primary extradural tumors are ordinarily discovered when they begin to compress the cord extrinsically. These consist predominantly of neoplasms of mesenchymal origin. Surgical extirpation can ordinarily control such tumors, and radiation therapy has virtually no part to play.

Metastases from various types of primary malignant neoplasms frequently affect the spinal cord. The incidence of such neoplastic manifestations is difficult to determine. These occur by involvement of the paravertebral soft tissues with invasion through the intervertebral foramina and infiltration between the dura itself and the vertebral canal. Once the metastatic process is within the vertebral canal it may extend in every direction including a circular fashion around the cord. Such metastatic invasion of the spinal canal is seen most frequently in cancer of the breast, bronchogenic carcinoma or hypernephroma. It is often observed in the lymphoma group, with Hodgkin's granuloma and lymphosarcoma.

Similar metastatic manifestations can also occur when metastases involve the body of vertebrae and break through the osseous barrier to extend into the vertebral canal. From the treatment standpoint, it is essential and most important that these lesions be suspected and identified early, so that adequate treatment can be established before permanent damage be inflicted on the cord, with resulting paraplegia. No matter how radiosensitive the tumor may be, it is imperative to perform a surgical decompression of the cord in all cases with paraplegic symptoms of 24-hour duration. Otherwise, permanent paraplegia is likely to settle.

When extradural pressure on the cord results from vertebral collapse due to metastatic involvement, immediate surgical decompression is imperative. In such cases the metastatic lesions are usually infiltrative in character and can rarely be removed completely by surgical excision at the time of decompression.

Palliative irradiation is indicated following surgical decompression of the cord. The plan of treatment will depend upon the nature and character of the metastatic process, and also its extent within the spinal canal as well as in the paravertebral region. Treatment planning must therefore be individualized after careful clinical assessment. It must also be adjusted or modified from time to time as required by the patient's condition. Some extradural metastatic lesions are secondary to certain carcinomas or sarcomas which may be radioresistant, and in such cases one must not expect a better response to radiation than the primary itself might give. Therefore the prognosis, the plan of treatment, and the radiation doses to be administered will be influenced by those factors. Extradural infiltration of the spinal canal and compression of the cord will often be relieved dramatically in the treatment of Hodgkin's or small cell lymphosarcoma following moderate doses of radiation therapy alone.

Enhancing effects may be obtained when radiation is associated with radiomimetic chemotherapeutic agents. Complete clinical evaluation of each case individually should be the most important and perhaps the only guide as to the plan of treatment either with radiation therapy alone or combined with palliative surgical procedures or chemotherapy.

SACROCOCCYGEAL CHORDOMA

Chordomas may be found in the sacrococcygeal region, but not frequently. In the series of 1322 cases of primary tumors involving the spinal canal, Slooff et al.[104] had 53 intraspinal chordomas and the majority were located in the sacral region. We have seen and treated only 4 cases arising from the sacrococcygeal area in our entire series of primary tumors involving the central nervous system. Recently, Kamerin, Potanos and Pool[52] presented 30 cases of chordomas of which 5 involved the sacrococcygeal area and 9 were found at other levels of the spinal column. Tumors in any of these locations invade the vertebral canal and press on the cord extradurally. The diagnosis is made at operation and subtotal removal is indicated first. Tumor doses must be high, but should rarely be less than 5000 to 6000 rads over a period of approximately 50 days using megavoltage radiation. The prognosis is not good. However, we have observed good palliative response in some of our cases. Kamerin and associates[52] have reported an average of 3 years of survival from the time of therapy.

MISCELLANEOUS BENIGN LESIONS

Syringomyelia

This is a benign condition located in the upper segment of the spinal cord and involving the ependymal canal which is dilated and usually filled with small cystic cavities. This process tends to expand into adjacent portions of the spinal cord. Syringomyelia is considered by many as a lesion of embryonal development. Gardner and Angel[39] have demonstrated that this is a developmental anomaly consisting of a diverticulum expanding from the central canal of the spinal cord which becomes dilated.

Syringomyelia must be differentiated from intramedullary tumors involving the cervical segment of the spinal cord. Slooff et al.[104] have stated that syringomyelia and cord tumors are frequently associated. They found such combination in 57.6 per cent of 33 cases of intramedullary tumors in which necropsy was done. They discovered 19 cases of syringomyelia among 33 intramedullary tumors.

The diagnosis of syringomyelia or hydromyelia will be facilitated in a certain proportion of the cases by various types of radiological examinations. McRae[76] has reviewed 55 cases diagnosed as syringomyelia and hydromyelia over a period of 30 years. He has analyzed the radiological evidence found in all cases, having divided them into two groups: 20 cases confirmed at operation or necropsy and 35 unproved cases. Scoliosis involving the cervical and thoracic segments of the spine, or either one alone, was found to be a predominant feature in approximately 85 per cent of all cases, either proved or unproved. Enlargement of the spinal canal both in the cervical and thoracic segments of the spine, or in either one alone, was observed in one half of the proved cases and in one quarter of the unproved. Bone changes about the foramen magnum and the upper segments of the spine were noted in approximately 20 per cent of the proved cases, and in a smaller proportion of the unproved cases. Myelograms in syringomyelia and hydromyelia revealed enlargement of the cord in 9 of 12 proven cases when oil was used, and in 14 of 23 unproved. The cord was found to be small at air myelography in all 6 patients subjected to this form of myelogram, some of whom had had a large cord at oil myelogram. A collapsing spinal cord seemed pathognomonic of syringomyelia. A differential diagnosis between syringomyelia and intramedullary tumor can be made radiologically in some cases, but if the two pathologic processes are associated together, surgical exploration may be indicated to arrive at a firm diagnosis.

From all the pathologic evidence accumulated regarding the pathogenesis of syringomyelia, it appears that this is a condition which is unlikely to be modified by radiation therapy. Gardner and Angel[39] have expressed the opinion that the symptoms of syringomyelia can be improved by surgical treatment in opening the obstructed foramen of Magendie. McIlroy and Richardson[74] have reviewed the records of 75 patients with syringomyelia and suggested that surgical treatment may be indicated in selected cases. They used x-ray therapy in 13 patients and in 9 the disease continued to progress despite irradiation, whereas relief of pain occurred in 1 patient. Dyke and Davidoff[30] have expressed the opinion that syringomyelia is a disease in which some cases appeared to respond favorably to roentgen therapy. However, they agreed that cures of the disease did not occur.

My own experience is limited to approximately 6 cases in which improvement of symptoms, particularly of pain, was evidenced following a short course of treatment with relatively small doses totalling in depth 1000 to 1200 r over a period of 10 to 15 days. Our follow-up is practically non-existent in this group of cases. Therefore I feel unable to offer any guidance in relation to the late results of treatment of syringomyelia by irradiation, which could be based upon my personal experience. However, I fail to visualize how radiation therapy could modify such pathological process. I have not treated patients with syringomyelia for a long time and I see no reason to modify this policy unless it might be solely for the palliation of pain.

Arachnoiditis

We have attempted to treat adhesive arachnoiditis with radiation in 4 cases. Total doses averaging 1500 to 1800 r depth dose have been administered at a slow rate over periods of 30 to 35 days. Our objective was to reduce the fibrotic adhesions existing between the surfaces of the arachnoid membrane. No definite evidence of improvement has been observed in the few cases that were treated.

12 Indications for Radiation Therapy in Certain Lesions Involving the Peripheral Nervous System

IRRADIATION OF NEOPLASTIC LESIONS INVOLVING NERVOUS TISSUE

Neuroblastomas

Malignant neoplastic lesions growing beyond the central nervous system consist of neuroblastomas almost exclusively. These are neurogenic tumors considered to be arising predominantly from the sympathetic nervous system. Neuroblastomas were found largely in the abdominal cavity at level of the adrenal glands in 38 of 81 cases reported by Phillips.[88] The thoracic cavity is a common site. Skeletal metastases were found on admission in 28 of the 86 cases reviewed by Koop and Hernandez.[59]

Neuroblastomas occur mostly in children. Among the 73 proven cases of Wittenborg,[118] 80 per cent of the patients were within the first 5 years of life.

Neuroblastomas have been known to undergo spontaneous regression, gradually becoming benign ganglioneuromas. No specific therapy was given in 28 of Wittenborg's patients and only 10 per cent survived over 3 years.

Neuroblastomas are considered radiosensitive, but many believe that the role of radiation therapy is not clear. With X-radiation alone, 6 of 22 patients or 27 per cent survived over 3 years in Wittenborg's series. The majority of cases in various reports have received postoperative irradiation. The doses used seem to differ substantially from one series to another. In Wittenborg's cases, 1400 to 1800 r were given in 7 to 10 days. Phillips referred to tumor doses of 2000 to 3000 r in 10 to 20 days. In the 165 cases reported by Williams,[117] the doses ranged from 1500 to 3500 r in 3 to 4 weeks.

Chemotherapy has been advocated and used alone or in combination

219

with other methods of treatment by some of the authors mentioned above and many others.

Results of treatment vary. Koop and Hernandez stated that, except for one, no patient with neuroblastoma who has been alive and well 14 months postoperatively died of the disease subsequently. In most series, 3-year survival rates vary between 22 to 36 per cent.

My experience in the management of patients with neuroblastomas is very limited. I have merely attempted to review the experience accumulated from large series published by others.

Neuromas and Neurofibromas

Peripheral nerves are recognized as structures which normally are rather radioresistant. This does not mean that nerve fibers are immune to radiation. When nerves are injured by irradiation, this seems to be by a process of demyelinization. The incidence of primary neoplasms arising from peripheral nerves is low. These tumors consist almost exclusively of slowly growing benign lesions, diagnosed histologically as neuromas, neurinomas, and neurofibromata. Peripheral nerve tumors are usually single and localized lesions. If they should be multiple, they nearly always are manifestations of generalized neurofibromatosis or von Recklinghausen's disease.

The management of these tumors, wherever they may be, is primarily a surgical problem. Radiation therapy should not be expected to induce regression of neuromas. At the most, there might be palliation of pain for a variable duration. This has been the experience of many observers through the years. Our last attempt at irradiation of a neuroma was entirely futile. A tumor dose of 6500 rads was delivered in 50 days to a large neuroma measuring approximately 12 cm. in diameter. This was a manifestation of generalized neurofibromatosis. The tumor was located in the posterior part of the pelvic cavity of a female patient and was therefore readily accessible for clinical observation. There was no appreciable beneficial effect on the tumor at any time during or after treatment.

Occasionally, small tumors involving a peripheral nerve may show partial regression under irradiation. Usually this is accompanied by relief of pain. Such radiation effects have been observed in 2 of our patients with recurrent neuromas in which a predominance of fibrous connective tissue reaction had been reported by the pathologist. These lesions were treated with tissue doses of 1000 to 1200 rads in small divided doses over a total period of 4 to 6 weeks. It is important to treat over a long protracted basis since our aim is to induce antifibrotic effect and not to cause more fibrosis. Total improvement may be appreciable 3 to 6 months only following completion of treatment.

Analgesic Effect of Radiation on Neoplastic Lesions

The analgesic effect of ionizing radiation on primary or secondary malignant tumors is often dramatic. Pain relief in patients with bone metastases or metastases infiltrating soft tissues unquestionably represents one of the most useful and beneficial utilizations of radiation for palliative purposes.

RADIATION EFFECTS ON NON-NEOPLASTIC NERVE CONDITIONS

Postherpetic Neuritis or Other Neuralgia

Palliative irradiation still has a place in the treatment of neuritis and severe neuralgia when this cannot be relieved satisfactorily by any other method. Patients should be so treated providing only that such treatment may not prevent or unduly delay investigation which might disclose some serious cause of pain which should be treated primarily and quite differently.

Postherpetic neuralgia is the most common neuritic condition that we are still treating nowadays with a reasonable amount of success. Severe neuralgia occurs in a minority of patients afflicted with herpes zoster. It is preferable to treat such neuralgia towards the end of an acute phase of herpes zoster, once it has become chronic and might persist indefinitely without irradiation. Radiation therapy directed over the corresponding nerve roots will often induce some degree of analgesic effect and at times relieve pain completely and permanently. It is wise to irradiate 1 or 2 nerve root levels above and below those apparently involved. Relief of pain may be observed towards the end of a course of treatment but improvement is slow, and complete results of treatment may not be fully appreciable until 2 to 3 months have elapsed from onset of treatment. Total relief of pain in postherpetic neuralgia may be anticipated in the majority of the acute cases and in a proportion of 40 to 50 per cent of patients in the chronic cases. Our plan of treatment usually consists of a total incident dose of 1500 to 1800 r, in divided doses of 150 r 3 times a week over a period of approximately 4 weeks. The tissue dose at level of the nerve roots varies between 1000 to 1200 rads. In a few cases the amount of peripheral scarring in the skin appears to be involving the nerve endings to such an extent that these have to be treated as well as the nerve roots. This is then treated on the same basis as that used for the treatment of keloids.

Trigeminal neuralgia has been treated in the same fashion on several occasions and with highly satisfactory results. The external radiation beam is then aimed to the gasserian ganglion and the emerging nerve roots.

Relief of Pain and/or Pruritus in Scars

Painful scars, associated or not with itchiness, may be quite distressing in some patients and these symptoms may be relieved completely by localized external irradiation. Such symptoms may manifest themselves with or without keloid formation. The radiobiologic objective is then to induce an antifibrotic reaction which will result in analgesia by freeing nerve endings and terminal nerve branches from constriction by scar tissue. This can be accomplished properly only if treatment is administered slowly and with doses which will not increase the existing fibrosis, but bring its regression. Fibrosis is a reversible reaction which may be either induced or reduced by ionizing radiation. Since tissue inflammation is a predominant factor in causing radiation fibrosis, it is important that any plan of treatment be such as to avoid causing inflammation in the treatment of painful scars. Single skin doses of 300 r at a time are administered every 2 or 3 weeks for a total of 4 or 5 treatments. Improvement usually begins to be appreciable, and sometimes relief of pain and itchiness is complete about the time the patient returns for the third treatment.

Bibliographic References

1. Abbott, K. H. and Kernohan, J. W.: Medulloblastomas; concerning the problems of spinal metastasis and malignancy; a report of six cases and discussion of the problems involved, Bull. Los Angeles Neurol. Soc., *8*, 1–10, 1943.
2. Arnold, A., Bailey, P. and Harvey, R. A.: Intolerance of primate brainstem and hypothalamus to conventional and high energy radiations, Neurology, *4*, 575–585, 1954.
3. Arnold, A., Bailey, P., Harvey, R. A. and Haas, L. L.: Application of betatron to treatment of brain tumors, Southern Med. J., *48*, 63–67, 1955.
4. Arnold, A., Bailey, P. and Laughlin, J. S.: Effects of betatron radiations on brain of primates, Neurology, *4*, 165–178, 1954.
5. Bachman, A. L. and Harris, W.: Roentgen therapy for pituitary adenoma; correlation of tumor dose with response in 64 cases, Radiology, *53*, 331–341, 1949.
6. Bailey, P. and Cushing, H.: Medulloblastoma cerebelli; common type of mid-cerebellar glioma of childhood, Arch. Neurol. & Psychiat., *14*, 192–224, 1925.
7. *A Classification of the Tumors of the Glioma Group on a Histogenetic Basis with a Correlated Study of Prognosis,* Philadelphia, J. B. Lippincott Co., p. 175, 1926.
8. Bailey, P.: *Intracranial Tumors,* 2d ed., Springfield, Charles C Thomas, p. 478, 1948.
9. Bercovici, B. and Ehrenfeld, E. N.: Non-puerperal galactorrhea, J. Obstet. Gynaec. Brit. Comm., *70*: 295–300, 1963.
10. Berger, E. and Elvidge, A. R.: Medulloblastomas and cerebellar sarcomas, *Proceedings of the 4th International Congress of Neuropathology, Munich, 1961.* (H. Jacob, Ed.), Stuttgart, Georg Thieme Verlag, pp. 364–373, 1962.
11. Boden, G.: Radiation myelitis of the cervical cord, Brit. J. Radiol., *21*, 464–469, 1948.
12. Radiation myelitis of the brain-stem, J. Fac. Radiologists, *2*, 79–94, 1950.
13. Bouchard, J.: Radiation therapy of malignant intracranial neoplasms, Progr. Radiat. Ther., *1*, 192–223, 1958.
14. Radiation therapy of intracranial neoplasms, *The Biology and Treatment of Intracranial Tumors,* (W. S. Fields and P. C. Sharkey, Eds). Springfield, Charles C Thomas, pp. 371–399, 1962.
15. Bouchard, J. and Peirce, C. B.: Radiation therapy in the management of neoplasms of the central nervous system, with a special note in regard to children: Twenty years' experience, 1939–1958, Amer. J. Roentgen., *84*, 610–628, 1960.
16. Buchanan, D.: Intracranial tumors in infancy and childhood. Amer. J. Surg., *93*, 935–940, 1957.

17. Cairns, H. and Russell, D. S.: Intracranial and spinal metastases in gliomas of the brain, Brain, *54*, 377–420, 1931.
18. Chao, J. H., Phillips, R., and Nickson, J. J.: Roentgen-ray therapy of cerebral metastases, Cancer, *7*, 682–689, 1954.
19. Chasmer, L. R., Robertson, D. C. and Farmer, A. W.: Irradiation fibrosarcoma, Plast. Reconstr. Surg., *20*, 55–61, 1957.
20. Clemente, C. D. and Holst, E. A.: Pathological changes in neurons, neuroglia and blood-brain barrier induced by x-irradiation of heads of monkeys, Arch. Neurol. & Psychiat., *71*, 66–79, 1954.
21. Concannon, J. P., Kramer, S. and Berry, R.: The extent of intracranial gliomata at autopsy and its relationship to techniques used in radiation therapy of brain tumors, Amer. J. Roentgen., *84*, 99–107, 1960.
22. Cone, W. V. and Elvidge, A.: Personal communication, 1958.
23. Correa, J. N. and Lampe, I.: The radiation treatment of pituitary adenomas. J. Neurosurg., *19*, 626–631, 1962.
24. Cutler, E. C., Sosman, M. C. and Vaughan, W. W.: The place of radiation in the treatment of cerebellar medulloblastomata, Amer. J. Roentgen., *35*, 429–453, 1936.
25. Dahlin, D. C. and MacCarty, C. S.: Chordoma; study of 59 cases, Cancer, *5*, 1170–1178, 1952.
26. Davidoff, L. M., Dyke, C. G., Elsberg, C. A. and Tarlov, I. M.: The effect of radiation applied directly to the brain and spinal cord; experimental investigations of Macacus rhesus monkeys, Radiology, *31*, 451–463, 1938.
27. Davis, L. and Davis, R. A.: Tumors of the hypophysis, *Principles of Neurological Surgery,* 5th ed., Philadelphia, W. B. Saunders Co., p. 608, 1963.
28. Dohan, F. C., Raventos, A., Boucot, N. and Rose, E.: Roentgen therapy in Cushing's syndrome without adrenocortical tumor. J. Clin. Endocr. *17*, 8–32, 1957.
29. Dugger, G. S., Stratford, J. G. and Bouchard, J.: Necrosis of brain following roentgen irradiation, Amer. J. Roentgen., *72*, 953–960, 1954.
30. Dyke, C. G., and Davidoff, L. M.: *Roentgen Treatment of Diseases of the Nervous System,* Philadelphia, Lea & Febiger, p. 198, 1942.
31. Elvidge, A., Penfield, W. and Cone, W.: The gliomas of the central nervous system. A study of two hundred and ten verified cases, Proceedings of the Association for Research in Nervous and Mental Diseases, *16*, 107–181, 145–154, 1935.
32. Elvidge, A. R. and Baldwin, M.: Clinical analysis of 88 cases of metastatic carcinoma involving central nervous system. J. Neurosurg., *6*, 495–502, 1949.
33. Feigin, I. H. and Gross, S. W.: Sarcoma arising in glioblastoma of brain, Amer. J. Path., *31*, 633–653, 1955.
34. Feindel, W., Yamamoto, Y. L., McRae, D. L. and Zanelli, J.: Contour brain scanning with iodine and mercury compounds for detection of intracranial tumors, Amer. J. Roentgen., *92*, 177–186, 1964.
35. Frankel, S. A., and German, W. J.: Glioblastoma multiforme: review of 219 cases with regard to natural history, pathology, diagnostic methods, and treatment, J. Neurosurg., *15*, 489–503, 1958.
36. Freid, J. R. and Davidoff, L. M.: Roentgen therapy of primary neoplasms of the brain, Radiology, *57*, 25–36, 1951.
37. French, L. A.: Some aspects of diagnosis and treatment of brain tumors in children, *The Biology and Treatment of Intracranial Tumors,* (W. S. Fields and P. C. Sharkey, Eds.), Springfield, Charles C Thomas, pp. 412–433, 1962.
38. Galluzzi, S., and Payne, P. M.: Brain metastases from primary bronchial carcinoma: a statistical study 741 necropies, Brit. J. Cancer, *10*, 408–414, 1956.
39. Gardner, W. J. and Angel, J.: The cause of syringomyelia and its surgical treatment, Cleveland Clin. Quart., *25*, 4–8, 1958.
40. German, W. J. and Flanigan, S.: Pituitary adenomas: A follow-up study of the Cushing series. Clin. Neurosurg., *10*, 72–81, 1964.
41. Goldberg, H. I., Heinz, J. M., and Taveras, J. M.: Preliminary experiences with thermography in neurological patients. VII Symposium Neuroradiologicum. Acta Radiol. (Diag.), In Press.

42. Godwin, J. T., Farr, L. E., Sweet, W. H. and Robertson, J. S.: Pathological study of eight patients with glioblastoma multiforme treated by neutron-capture therapy using boron, 10, Cancer, 8, 601–615, 1955.
43. Henderson, W. R.: The pituitary adenomata. A follow-up of the surgical results in 338 cases, Brit. J. Surg., 26, 811–921, 1939.
44. Ho. J. H. C.: Personal communication, 1966.
45. Horrax, G.: Benign (favorable) types of brain tumor; end results (up to 20 years), with statistics of mortality and useful survival, New Eng. J. Med., 250, 981–984, 1954.
46. Treatment of pituitary adenomas; surgery versus radiation, Arch. Neur. Psychiat. 79, 1–6, 1958.
47. Ingraham, F. D. and Matson, D. D.: Neurosurgery of Infancy and Childhood, Springfield, Charles C Thomas, pp. 259–269, 1954.
48. Jones, A.: Orbital X-ray therapy of progressive exophthalmos, Brit. J. Radiol., 24, 637–646, 1951.
49. Supervoltage X-ray therapy of intracranial tumors, Ann. Roy. Coll. Surg. Engl., 27, 310–354, 1960.
50. Kageyama, N.: Communication of Zimmerman, H. N., The Biology and Treatment of Intracranial Tumors, (W. S. Fields and P. C. Sharkey, Eds.), Springfield, Charles C Thomas, pp. 64–69, 1962.
51. Kahn, E. A., Bassett, R. C., Schneider, R. C. and Crosby, E. C.: Correlative Neurosurgery, Springfield, Charles C Thomas, pp. 214–231, 1955.
52. Kamerin, R. P., Potanos, J. N. and Pool, J. L.: An evaluation of the diagnosis and treatment of chordoma, J. Neurol. Neurosurg. Psychiat., 27, 157–165, 1964.
53. Kelly, K. H., Felsted, E. T., Brown, R. F., Ortega, P., Bierman, H. R., Low-Beer, B. V. A. and Shimkin, M. G.: Irradiation of the normal human hypophysis in malignancy: report of 3 cases receiving 8,100–10,000 r tissue dose to the pituitary glands. J. Nat. Cancer Inst., 11, 967–983, 1951.
54. Kernohan, J. W., Woltman, H. W. and Adson, A. W.: Intramedullary tumors of the spinal cord; review of 51 cases, with attempt at histologic classification, Arch. Neurol. & Psychiat., 25, 679–701, 1931.
55. Kernohan, J. W., Mabon, R. F., Svien, H. J., and Adson, A. W.: A simplified classification of the gliomas, Proc. Staff Meet. Mayo Clin., 24, 71–75, 1949.
56. Kernohan, J. W. and Uihlein, A.: Sarcomas of the Brain, Springfield, Charles C Thomas, pp. 25–29, 120–153, 154–169, 1962.
57. Kerr, H. D., Irradiation of pituitary tumors, Amer. J. Roentgen., 60, 348–359, 1948.
58. Kerr, F. W. L., Schwartz, H. G. and Seaman, W. B.: Experimental effects of radioactive colloidal gold in subarachnoid space; clinical application in treating brain tumor, Arch. Surg., 69, 694–706, 1954.
59. Koop, C. E. and Hernandez, J. R.: Neuroblastoma: experience with 100 cases in children, Surgery, 56, 726–733, 1964.
60. Kramer, S., McKissock, W. and Concannon, J. P.: Craniopharyngiomas. Treatment by combined surgery and radiation therapy, J. Neurosurg., 18, 217–226, 1961.
61. Kricheff, I. I., Becker, M., Schneck, S. A. and Taveras, J. M.: Intracranial ependymomas. A Study of survival in 65 cases treated by surgery and irradiation, Amer. J. Roentgen., 91, 167–175, 1964.
62. Kurland, L. T.: The frequency of intracranial and intraspinal neoplasms in the resident population of Rochester, Minnesota, J. Neurosurg., 15, 627–641, 1958.
63. Kurland, L. T., Myrianthopoulos, N. C. and Lessel, S.: Epidemiologic and genetic considerations of intracranial neoplasms, The Biology and Treatment of Intracranial Tumors, (W. S. Fields and P. C. Sharkey, Eds.), Springfield, Charles C Thomas, pp. 5–48, 1962.
64. Lampe, I. and MacIntyre, R. S.: Experiences in the radiation therapy of medulloblastoma of the cerebellum. Amer. J. Roentgen., 71, 659–668, 1954.
65. Lampe, I.: Radiation tolerance of the central nervous system, Progr. Radiat. Ther., 1, 224–236, 1958.

66. Lawrence, J. H. and Tobias, C. A.: Heavy particles in medicine, *Progress in Atomic Medicine,* (J. H. Lawrence, Ed.), New York, Grune & Stratton, pp. 127–143, 1965.
67. Levy, L. F. and Elvidge, A. R.: Astrocytoma of the brain and spinal cord; a review of 176 cases, 1940–1949, J. Neurosurg., *13,* 413–443, 1956.
68. Lindgren, M.: On tolerance of brain tissue and sensitivity of brain tumors to irradiation, Acta Radiol., Supp. *170,* 1–73, 1958.
69. Llewellyn, R. C. and Creech, O., Jr.: Perfusion for cerebral tumors, *The Biology and Treatment of Intracranial Tumors,* (W. S. Fields and P. C. Sharkey, Eds.), Springfield, Charles C Thomas, pp. 400–411, 1962.
70. Lowenberg-Scharenberg, K. and Bassett, R. C.: Amyloid degeneration of human brain following x-ray therapy, J. Neuropath. Exp. Neurol., *9,* 93–102, 1950.
71. Luse, S. A.: Electron microscopy of brain tumors, *The Biology and Treatment of Intracranial Tumors,* (W. S. Fields and P. C. Sharkey, Eds.), Springfield, Charles C Thomas, pp. 75–103, 1962.
72. MacCarty, C. S.: Results of the surgical management of glial tumors of the brain, *The Biology and Treatment of Intracranial Tumors,* (W. S. Fields and P. C. Sharkey, Eds.), Springfield, Charles C Thomas, pp. 434–456, 1962.
73. Mann, I., Yates, P. C. and Ainslie, J. P.: Unusual case of double primary orbital tumor, Brit. J. Ophthal., *37,* 758–762, 1953.
74. McIlroy, W. J. and Richardson, J. C.: Syringomyelia: a clinical review of 75 cases, Canad. Med. Ass. J., *93,* 731–734, 1965.
75. McRae, D. L. and Elliott, A. W.: Radiological aspects of cerebellar astrocytomas and medulloblastomas, Acta Radiol., *50,* 52–66, 1958.
76. McRae, D. L.: Personal communication, 1966.
77. McWhirter, R. and Dott, N. M.: Tumors of the brain and spinal cord. *British Practice in Radiotherapy,* (E. R. Carling, B. W. Windeyer and D. W. Smithers, Eds.), London, Butterworth & Co. Ltd., pp. 330–346, 1955.
78. Merriam, G. R. and Focht, E. F.: Radiation cataracts and relationship to dose, Amer. J. Roentgen., *77,* 759–785, 1957.
79. Mitchell, J. S.: *Studies in Radiotherapeutics,* Cambridge, Massachusetts, Harvard University Press, pp. 212–221, 1960.
80. Nessa, C. B.: Effect of treatment of brain tumors with roentgen rays, Radiology, *31,* 670–677, 1938.
81. Noetzli, M. and Malamud, N.: Postirradiation fibrosarcoma of the brain, Cancer, *15,* 617–622, 1962.
82. Paterson, E. and Farr, R. F.: Cerebellar medulloblastoma: treatment by irradiation of whole central nervous system. Acta Radiol., *39,* 323–336, 1953.
83. Paterson, R.: *The Treatment of Malignant Disease by Radiotherapy,* 2d ed., London, Edward Arnold Ltd., pp. 451–463, 1963.
84. Peirce, C. B., Cone, W. V., Bouchard, J. and Lewis, R. C.: Medulloblastoma: non-operative management with roentgen therapy after aspiration biopsy, Radiology, *52,* 621–632, 1949.
85. Peirce, C. B. and Bouchard, J.: Role of radiation therapy in the control of malignant neoplasms of the brain and brain stem, Radiology, *55,* 337–342, 1950.
86. Penfield, W. and Feindel, W.: Medulloblastoma of cerebellum, with survival for 17 years, Arch. Neurol. Psychiat., *57,* 481–484, 1947.
87. Pennybacker, J. and Russell, D. S.: Necrosis of the brain due to radiation therapy; clinical and pathological observations, J. Neurol., Neurosurg. & Psychiat., *11,* 183–198, 1948.
88. Phillips, R.: Neuroblastoma, Ann. Roy. Coll. Surg. Eng., *12,* 29–48, 1953.
89. Pool, J. L., Ransohoff, J. and Correll, J. W.: The treatment of malignant brain tumors, primary and metastatic, New York J. Med., *57,* 3983–3988, 1957.
90. Poppen, J. L.: Surgical treatment of extracerebral intracranial tumors, *The Biology and Treatment of Intracranial Tumors,* (W. S. Fields and P. C. Sharkey, Eds.), Springfield, Charles C Thomas, pp. 457–480, 1962.
91. Raimondi, A. J.: The localization of risa in human gliomas. An electron-microscopic study. VII Symposium Neuroadiologicum, Acta Radiol. (Diag.), In Press.

92. Rasmussen, T. B., Kernohan, J. W. and Adson, A. W.: Pathologic classification, with surgical consideration, of intraspinal tumors, Ann. Surg., *3*, 513–530, 1940.
93. Rasmussen, T., Harper, P. V. and Kennedy, T.: The use of beta ray point source for destruction of the hypophysis, Surg. Forum, *4*, 681–686, 1953.
94. Ray, B. S. and Horwith, M.: Surgical treatment of acromegaly, Clin. Neurosurg., *10*, 31–59, 1964.
95. Reynolds, L.: Newer investigations of radiation effects and their clinical applications, Amer. J. Roentgen., *55*, 135–152, 1946.
96. Richards, P., McKissock, W.: Intracranial metastases, Brit. Med. J. *1*, 15–18, 1963.
97. Richmond, J. J.: Radiotherapy of intracranial tumors in children, J. Fac. Radiologists, *4*, 180–189, 1953.
98. Discussion on pituitary tumors: the role of radiotherapy, Proc. Roy. Soc. Med., *51*, 911–914, 1958.
99. Ringertz, N. and Reymond, A.: Ependymomas and choroid plexus papillomas. J. Neuropath. Exp. Neurol., *8*, 355–380, 1949.
100. Ringertz, N.: "Grading" of gliomas, Acta Path. Microbiol. Scand., *27*, 51–64, 1950.
101. Rovit, R. L. and Berry, R.: Cushing's syndrome and the hypophysis. A re-evaluation of pituitary tumors and hyperadrenalism, J. Neurosurg., *23*, 270–295, 1965.
102. Russell, D. S., Wilson, C. W. and Tansley, K.: Experimental radio-necrosis of the brain in rabbits, J. Neurol., Neurosurg. Psychiat., *12*, 187–195, 1949.
103. Russell, D. S. and Rubinstein, L. J.: *Pathology of Tumors of the Nervous System*, 2nd. ed., London, E. Arnold Ltd., pp. 60–61, 1963.
104. Slooff, J. L., Kernohan, J. W. and MacCarty, C. S.: *Primary Intramedullary Tumors of the Spinal Cord and Filum Terminale*, Philadelphia, W. B. Saunders Co., p. 255, 1964.
105. Sheline, G. E., Boldrey, E. B. and Phillips, T. L.: Chromophobe adenomas of the pituitary gland, Amer. J. Roentgen., *92*, 160–173, 1964.
106. Smith, R. A., Lampe, I. and Kahn, E. A.: The prognosis of medulloblastoma in children, J. Neurosurg., *18*, 91–97, 1961.
107. Sosman, M. C.: Roentgen therapy of pituitary adenomas, J. A. M. A., *113*, 1282–1285, 1939.
108. Cushing's disease—pituitary basophilism, Amer. J. Roentgen., *62*, 1–32, 1949.
109. Störtebecker, T. P.: Metastatic tumors of the brain from a neurological point of view; follow-up study of 158 cases, J. Neurosurg., *11*, 84–111, 1954.
110. Svien, H. J., Gates, E. M. and Kernohan, J. W.: Spinal subarachnoid implantation associated with ependymoma, Arch. Neurol. Psychiat., *62*, 847–856, 1949.
111. Talairach, J., Ruggiero, G., Aboulker, J. and David, M.: New method of treatment of inoperable brain tumor by stereotaxic implantation of radioactive gold—preliminary report, Brit. J. Radiol., *28*, 62–74, 1955.
112. Talairach, J., Szikla, G., Bonis, A., Tournoux, P., Bancaud, J., Mempel, E.: Radiothérapie interstitielle pour exophtalmie maligne et syndrome de Cushing d'origine haute, Presse Méd, *70*, 1399–1402, 1449–1451, 1962.
113. Terry, R. D., Hyams, V. J. and Davidoff, L. M.: Combined non metastasizing fibrosarcoma and chromophobe tumor of the pituitary, Cancer, *12*, 791–798, 1959.
114. Unger, S. M. and Roswit, B.: Restoration of the sella turcica after treatment of pituitary adenomas, Amer. J. Roentgen., *81*, 967–971, 1959.
115. Vaeth, J. M.: Radiation-induced myelitis, Progr. Radiat. Ther., *3*, 16–24, 1965.
116. Wachowski, T. J. and Chenault, H.: Degenerative effects of large doses of roentgen rays on the human brain, Radiology, *45*, 227–246, 1945.
117. Williams, I. G.: The treatment of malignant disease in childhood, Proc. Roy. Soc. Med., *58*, 609–614, 1965.
118. Wittenborg, M. H.: Roentgen therapy in neuroblastoma, Radiology, *54*, 679–687, 1950.

119. Woltman, H. W., Kernohan, J. W., Adson, A. W. and Craig, W. M.: Intramedullary tumors of spinal cord gliomas of intradural portion of filum terminale; fate of patients who have these tumors, Arch. Neurol. Psychiat., *65*, 378–395, 1951.
120. Wood, E. H. and Himadi, G. M.: Chordomas: roentgenologic study of 16 cases previously unreported, Radiology, *54*, 706–716, 1950.
121. Wood, E. H., Berne, A. S. and Taveras, J. M.: The value of radiation therapy in the management of intrinsic tumors of the spinal cord, Radiology, *63*, 11–24, 1954.
122. Zimmerman, H. M., and Arnold, H.: Experimental brain tumors; tumors produced with Benzpyrene, Amer. J. Path., *19*, 939–955, 1943.
123. Zimmerman, H. M., Netsky, M. G. and Davidoff, L. M.: *Atlas of Tumors of the Nervous System*, Philadelphia, Lea & Febiger, p. 191, 1956.
124. Zimmerman, H. M.: The natural history of intracranial neoplasms, with special reference to the gliomas, Amer. J. Surg., *93*, 913–924, 1957.
125. Personal communication, 1961.
126. Experimental brain tumors. *The Biology and Treatment of Intracranial Tumors*, (W. S. Fields and P. C. Sharkey, Eds.), Springfield, Charles C Thomas, pp. 49–74, 1962.
127. Zulch, K. J.: The present state of the classification of intracranial tumors and its value for the neurosurgeon, *The Biology and Treatment of Intracranial Tumors*, (W. S. Fields and P. C. Sharkey, Eds.), Springfield, Charles C Thomas, pp. 157–177, 1962.
128. Neurinomas, meningiomas, and related tumors, *The Biology and Treatment of Intracranial Tumors*, (W. S. Fields and P. C. Sharkey, Eds.), Springfield, Charles C Thomas, pp. 218–247, 1962.

index

229